INSTRUCTOR'S MANUAL TO ACCOMPANY
AN ILLUSTRATED GUIDE TO VETERINARY MEDICAL TERMINOLOGY

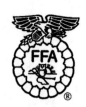

Join us on the web at
agriculture.delmar.com

INSTRUCTOR'S MANUAL TO ACCOMPANY
AN ILLUSTRATED GUIDE TO VETERINARY MEDICAL TERMINOLOGY

THIRD EDITION

Janet Amundson Romich, DVM, MS

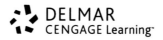

DELMAR
CENGAGE Learning

Australia • Brazil • Japan • Korea • Mexico • Singapore • Spain • United Kingdom • United States

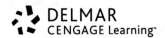
DELMAR
CENGAGE Learning™

Instructor's Manual to Accompany An Illustrated Guide to Veterinary Medical Terminology, Third Edition
Janet Amundson Romich

Vice President, Career and Professional
  Editorial: Dave Garza

Director of Learning Solutions: Matthew Kane

Acquisitions Editor: Benjamin Penner

Managing Editor: Marah Bellegarde

Senior Product Manager: Darcy M. Scelsi

Editorial Assistant: Scott Royael

Vice President, Career and Professional
  Marketing: Jennifer McAvey

Marketing Director: Debbie Yarnell

Marketing Manager: Erin Brennan

Marketing Coordinator: Jonathan Sheehan

Production Director: Carolyn Miller

Production Manager: Andrew Crouth

Senior Content Project Manager:
  Elizabeth C. Hough

Art Director: David Arsenault

Technology Project Manager: Benjamin Knapp

For product information and technology assistance, contact us at
Professional & Career Group Customer Support, 1-800-648-7450

For permission to use material from this text or product,
submit all requests online at **www.cengage.com/permissions**
Further permissions questions can be e-mailed to
permissionrequest@cengage.com

ISBN-13: 978-1-4354-2013-7

ISBN-10: 1-4354-2013-6

Delmar
5 Maxwell Drive
Clifton Park, NY 12065-2919
USA

Cengage Learning products are represented in Canada by Nelson Education, Ltd.

For your lifelong learning solutions, visit **www.delmar.cengage.com**

Visit our corporate website at **www.cengage.com**

Notice to the Reader

Publisher does not warrant or guarantee any of the products described herein or perform any independent analysis in connection with any of the product information contained herein. Publisher does not assume, and expressly disclaims, any obligation to obtain and include information other than that provided to it by the manufacturer. The reader is expressly warned to consider and adopt all safety precautions that might be indicated by the activities described herein and to avoid all potential hazards. By following the instructions contained herein, the reader willingly assumes all risks in connection with such instructions. The publisher makes no representations or warranties of any kind, including but not limited to, the warranties of fitness for particular purpose or merchantability, nor are any such representations implied with respect to the material set forth herein, and the publisher takes no responsibility with respect to such material. The publisher shall not be liable for any special, consequential, or exemplary damages resulting, in whole or part, from the readers' use of, or reliance upon, this material.

Printed in the United States of America
  1 2 3 4 5   14 13 12 11 10

ED006

CONTENTS

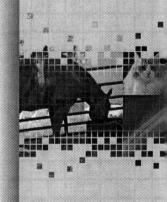

PART I

[TEACHING TIPS]

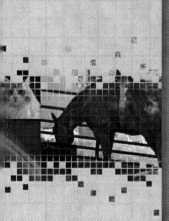

Teaching veterinary medical terminology is no different from teaching other subjects in that instructors need to consider the fact that students learn differently. Some students learn by doing (kinesthetic learners); others, by hearing (auditory learners); and still others, by seeing (visual learners). It is important to recognize that most students learn through a combination of these styles, so using varied teaching techniques that address the different learning styles will help your students learn and retain information better.

Your goal in planning should be to have students actively participate in class and to fully involve as many senses as possible. This teaching format accommodates different learning styles, aids in holding students' attention, and makes the class more interesting for students and for you.

Generous use of a chalkboard, transparencies, or computer-based presentation programs help students see a medical term while it is being discussed. Pronouncing the term while presenting it visually helps students associate the two. As students progress in their understanding of medical terminology, it is helpful to pronounce the term and have students define it both in written and oral form. Remember that on the job, students will not always see the medical term written down so that they can analyze it. It is similar to learning a foreign language. Seeing and analyzing foreign words is valuable in the learning stages, but using a foreign language in conversation and communication is the ultimate goal. One would not want a student who took French only to be able to conjugate verbs and not be able to order food at a French restaurant. Medical terminology works the same way. Having students listen to a description of a case history and then asking them what is happening is very valuable. Sometimes, you may need to go through the history very slowly and stop at key words; but this helps students retain medical terms and observe how those terms are used in context, and it improves students' listening skills.

Aids for developing good study skills and habits are also worthwhile to introduce in medical terminology courses. Using multiple colors of chalks or markers helps students group terms together and associate them with each other. For example, cardiovascular terms may be written in red, and urinary terms may be written in yellow. Then when you present the term *hematuria,*

1

you can write *hemat/o* in red and *-uria* in yellow. Because red is a darker color than yellow, *hematuria* will present itself as yellow urine that has become discolored with red blood. Not all samples of hematuria are red to the naked eye, but it does serve as a visual clue. When presenting the term *uremia*, *ur/o* may be written in yellow and *-emia* written in red. Since red is a darker color than yellow, the blood remains red but now has a yellow substance (urine or waste products) in it. Because students typically confuse the terms *hematuria* and *uremia*, it is important to give them as many memory tools as possible.

Word parts can also be written in different colors. Prefixes may be one color, root words another color, and suffixes still another color. If word parts are presented in three columns, students can mix and match them to make up their own terms. Even during the first few days of class, you will be amazed at how many accurate words students make.

For students who learn better by doing, it is helpful to work with instructors of other courses to have them use medical terms in their classes. To reinforce their learning of directional terms, students should be using those terms in animal handling classes. Live animals may be brought to the classroom for demonstrating directional terms. While holding an animal, students may be quizzed on directional terms and planes of the body. Videotapes of actual medical cases and reenactment of those cases also help reinforce words from a particular body system. Students usually can come up with other hands-on activities as well.

THE SUPPORTIVE CLASSROOM

Students who are comfortable in their environment do better in their studies, and an important factor in students' success is their knowing that the classroom provides a supportive environment. In this setting, students should feel free to learn without fear of ridicule or teasing. No question or comment is "stupid" during the learning process. The manner in which you structure class activities helps create such a setting.

The use of teams and team activities in class gives students a chance to work together to solve problems and does not make weaker students stand out from stronger students. Most veterinary clinics are based on the team approach, and this is a good skill for students to develop early in their career. Some instructors believe that the team approach divides the class and forms cliques, but when handled correctly, that problem can be avoided. It is helpful to rotate groups throughout the semester. Assigning partners or groups is another way to get students to work with different classmates during the course. The assigning of captains and team players often help the teams focus on the activity because everyone has his or her own responsibilities. The competition that arises between teams may motivate students to perform better.

Many class activities require students to work individually. Although some students are not comfortable working by themselves, a supportive atmosphere will help students become more confident in their abilities. Sometimes it takes a while for students to become comfortable in this setting, but when they do, they begin to ask questions and participate in discussions. This is a great feeling for you and the students.

Peer teaching is another way to help students learn and to build their self-confidence. Students may tutor each other in small groups or "team teach" with you on certain topics. If one student is having difficulty grasping the concept of medical word parts, another student can provide help and may provide a new suggestion for remembering the material. In some class periods, you can assign students a medical term from a specific unit and ask them to think of a way to remember it. Then go around the classroom asking students how they remember the term. By sharing information, a student does not have to provide all of the answers for every term, but rather an answer for just one or two terms. Students usually come up with creative ways to remember a term. Peer teaching also gets students comfortable with talking and studying outside of class.

Most instructors of medical terminology have developed mnemonics or other memory aids to help students remember difficult information. You can use your creativity and sense of humor when creating these learning aids. Flash cards get students to "play" with medical terms. Students also find rhyming phrases and letter association to be effective at remembering medical terms. For example, students tend to confuse the choana and the cloaca of birds. If you tell students that the term with the *h* is closer to the head (*h* and *h*), they usually can differentiate the two. The aorta is an artery because both begin with *a*. The list goes on and on.

GOALS OF TEACHING MEDICAL TERMINOLOGY

Students must understand what is expected of them in a medical terminology course. Without knowing the expected outcomes students become frustrated or overwhelmed with what is expected of them. They also need to know how they will be evaluated. When presented with all of the facts prior to starting the course, students can focus on learning the medical terms and not on trying to figure out the instructor's expectations.

In a medical terminology course, students must master the following foundation knowledge:

- Describe the types of medical word parts and state how each type is used.
- Spell and define commonly used medical word parts.
- State the rules for use of the combining vowel in medical terminology.

- Demonstrate the use of a medical dictionary in finding and defining medical terms.
- Describe the major body systems, their organs, and their functions.

In a medical terminology course, students are expected to master these competencies or end results:

- Recognize, pronounce, spell, and define commonly used medical terms relating to the diagnosis, pathology, and treatment of each body system.
- Given the definition of a medical term made up of medical word parts, find the term and spell and pronounce it correctly.
- Given an unfamiliar medical term that can be broken down into medical word parts, provide a reasonable definition.
- Use a medical dictionary and similar reference materials to find the meaning of medical terms and commonly used abbreviations.

EVALUATION CRITERIA

To evaluate competency in medical terminology, take into consideration the method of assessment, the decision as to whether the use of a medical dictionary is permitted, the time students have to complete the test, the passing score, and the number of attempts students are permitted.

Methods of Evaluation

A written test is the most efficient way to evaluate medical terminology competencies in a classroom setting. Almost any type of question can be used.

To test spelling, you can include a brief dictation section at the beginning of the test. Then students are allowed to proceed through the rest of the test at their own pace.

A written test does not assess the pronunciation of terms. If time permits, you can test students on this by listening to each student pronounce a list of, for example, 10 terms. Or, you can evaluate their pronunciation throughout the course in a less formal manner.

Use of a Medical Dictionary

Because the ability to use a medical dictionary is one of the competencies being tested, you should include questions to assess this skill.

Some instructors do not advocate the use of a dictionary because they fear students will not take time to study when they know they can look up answers. However, because students have a certain amount of time to complete the test, using a dictionary is a limited advantage. An alternative is to allow the use of a dictionary for only one section of the test that is given on a separate piece of paper. After you provide students with a specific time frame, they can complete this part of the test first. Or, you can assess dictionary use through a quiz on a separate day.

If you still oppose the use of a dictionary on test day, include questions that test its use; for example, "Under what dictionary heading would you find *bovine viral diarrhea*?"

Time Limit

A time limit is particularly important if students are allowed to use a medical dictionary. The amount of time allocated for a test depends on the number of items on the test and their format. Students should be informed of the time limit before the test session.

Point Value

You should provide the point value of each test item so that students know which questions are more important and thus are weighted heavier. You also should give the total points for a section so that students are aware of how many points each section or question type is worth.

Passing Score

In the ideal world, only 100 percent performance by a medical health professional is acceptable. However, in an academic setting, the level of a passing score is usually determined by school policy.

Number of Attempts Permitted

Some instructors permit only one attempt to demonstrate a competency. This relates to the theory that in the workplace, there is only one opportunity to "get it right."

Other instructors allow more than one attempt for certain skills. These instructors believe that students should increase their skill with each attempt; therefore, if a student wants to improve a grade, he or she should be allowed to retest. However, there is usually some point penalty for each retest. This means that even if a student answers all of the questions correctly on a retest, the highest possible score is less than 100.

TEST CONSTRUCTION

The first step in test construction is to review your course goals and determine what you are testing for. Computerized test banks are useful, but unless you follow the textbook rigidly, some of the questions may not relate to the material you emphasized. Ask yourself what you want students to remember today, remember at the end of the course, remember on the job, and remember five years from now. A good balance of those types of questions will result in a good test.

The skills being tested in a medical terminology course are cognitive; most written question formats are acceptable for testing. The primary exception is the use of true/false or other questions that allow only two answer choices, automatically giving students a 50-50 chance of guessing correctly.

Make sure that any test you give is free from spelling and grammatical errors. When being tested for language skills, students are easily confused by spelling errors because they think these are a trick to make sure they are reading for detail. Grammatical errors often produce questions in which students cannot determine what is being asked. Thus, they cannot demonstrate their knowledge.

Question Types

Fill in the Blank

These types of questions are effective for testing students' ability to read a definition and supply the term. Spelling can also be checked with this type of question. Make sure students know beforehand that they must spell the term correctly to receive full credit. The disadvantage is that these questions take longer to correct.

Multiple Choice

These types of questions can be adapted to most topics and testing situations. Remember that there are various levels of multiple choice questions, ranging from a basic level (basically testing memorization) to a more advanced level (testing logic and reasoning skills). Questions on a variety of levels should be included.

Tips for Writing Multiple Choice Questions

The Questions

- The question or stem is an introductory statement or question to which students must respond. The stem should be as short and simple as possible. You are testing students' comprehension, not their ability to decipher complex questions.
- The question may be in the form of a direct question; for example, "What is the medical term for increased urination?" This is an effective format.
- The question may be in the form of an incomplete sentence; for example, "Toward the head is called _____." This is also an effective format.
- The question may be in the form of a fill-in-the-blank question. This is an acceptable alternative to the direct question and incomplete sentence; for example, "Hematemesis means _____ blood."
- The question may be in the form of a negatively worded question. This type of question is more difficult because students must interpret the question and then find the

answer; for example, "Which of the following is not a medical term for feces?"

The Answers

- The answers or choices are one correct answer and the distractors (incorrect answers). An effective multiple choice question has four possible answers. Fewer choices allow students to guess more easily. More choices increase the difficulty of the question.
- If the question or stem is written as an incomplete sentence, the answers must flow to complete the sentence.
- Verb tense in the answer should agree with that of the question. Any change in verb tense will give students a clue that a particular answer is made up.
- All distractors should be believable and fit with the question format.
- All answers should be of approximately equal length.
- The answers should be as short as possible.
- Any term or phrase that appears in all of the answers probably should be moved to the question.
- The answers should be arranged in alphabetical or logical order so that the answers proceed from shortest to longest.
- If one of the answers is "some of the above choices" (i.e., A and B are correct), it should be the last choice if another answer is "all of the above." That way students are not confused as to whether the choice indicating that A and B are correct is included in the choice indicating all of the above.

Matching

These types of questions have some items in one column and the answers for those items in another column. Students match the questions and answers from both columns. Matching questions are effective when a series of similar items are challenging to differentiate. For example, types of muscle movements or projections on bones are well suited for matching questions. If there are equal numbers of items in both columns, the questions are easier for students. If there are unequal numbers of items in both columns or if some of the choices can be used more than once, the questions are more difficult.

Labeling

These types of questions require students to identify items on a diagram and supply the answer. Labeling questions are frequently used for anatomy and physiology questions. Labeling of directional terms is also examined effectively with this technique. When using this type of question, make sure the illustration is free of distractions and the parts being questioned are clear.

COURSE PLANNING SUGGESTIONS

Developing a Syllabus

Preparation of the syllabus is the beginning point of your planning process. The syllabus is a contract between you and your students and describes what is to be taught, when it will be taught, and what method of presentation will be used. It also should include the tentative dates of quizzes and examinations as well as assignment due dates. A syllabus should include the course name and number, course goal statement, your name and office (including room number, phone number, and e-mail address), time and days the course meets, and attendance policy (if you so choose). The body of the syllabus should include the following:

- Required and/or recommended texts
- Materials students need for class
- Teaching methods that will be used (required reading and exercises to be done before class, format of class time, etc.)
- Quizzes and examinations (and what each will cover)
- Assessment methods (including point assignment)

Developing a Course Outline

The course outline details what is to be covered during each week of the course. It also states the assignments students are expected to complete in preparation for class, identifies when tests are scheduled, and helps ensure that all class sections cover the same information.

Each student should receive a copy of the syllabus and the course outline at the beginning of the course. Based on this information, students know what is expected of them and when it is expected, leaving no room for surprises or excuses.

Developing an effective syllabus and course outline allows you to see how much material can be covered. For example, *An Illustrated Guide to Veterinary Medical Terminology*, 3E, has 23 chapters. Most schools do not have 23-week courses, so you must decide how and when to present the material. For most instructors, chapters 18 through 23 will be supplements to other chapters. Some body system chapters are longer than others, and you need to decide whether any chapters can be combined and covered in one week. An example syllabus is as follows:

Week 1: Chapter 1 and begin Chapter 2
Week 2: Finish Chapter 2
Week 3: Chapter 3
Week 4: Chapters 4 and 5
Examination

Week 5: Chapter 6
Week 6: Chapter 7
Week 7: Chapter 8
Week 8: Chapter 9
Examination

Week 9: Chapters 10 and 11
Week 10: Chapter 12
Week 11: Chapter 13
Week 12: Chapters 14 and 15
Examination

Week 13: Chapter 16
Week 14: Chapter 17
Week 15: Review material (using Chapters 18–23 as a guide)
Week 16: Review material (using Chapters 18–23 as a guide)
Final Examination

In the course outline, reading assignments, optional assignments, and student practice exercises can be assigned. This further clarifies the expectations that students must meet to complete the course successfully.

PART II

[TEACHING AIDS]

This section includes support materials that students may find helpful in learning veterinary medical terminology.

STUDENT STUDY SUGGESTIONS

1. Study the text and complete the review exercises at the end of each chapter.
2. Do not try to learn all of the words in one night (especially before a test).
3. Study regularly—20 to 30 minutes each day in *review* is helpful.
4. Do not be overwhelmed by the amount of material. At some point, it will seem as though the word parts are reshuffled parts that you already know.
5. Use activity cards. Carry them with you and use them when you have a few free minutes.
6. Listen to audio recordings.
7. Say the words and definitions aloud.
8. Write the words and their definitions.
9. Form a study group or pair to quiz each other.
10. Work medical terminology puzzles or do fun activities to keep the information at your fingertips.

FLASH CARDS

Flash cards have always served as an effective study tool for learning medical terms. Having students make the cards themselves helped them learn the words as they prepared the cards, but it was a time-consuming project that sometimes hindered the time students spent studying. Making grid sheets for students to photocopy is one way instructors can help students spend less time making the cards and more time studying them.

The StudyWARE™ CD that accompanies the text contains electronic flash cards and audio pronunciations. Students can quiz themselves on medical

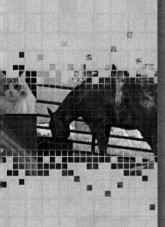

terms or medical definitions. The program supplements the text by quizzing students on the most commonly used terms from *An Illustrated Guide to Veterinary Medical Terminology*, 3E. The program is organized to correlate to the chapters in the text. The program includes approximately 5,000 words, so it serves as a good resource for students.

Auditory Learning

The audio library on the StudyWARE™ CD is a versatile teaching aid for use in the classroom, independent study, or distance education programs. Suggestions for using the audio include the following:

- Have students listen to the term in the audio library as they work through the chapters in the text. Students often get frustrated when they cannot pronounce a term and when they have difficulty with pronunciation keys or need positive reinforcement of the term's pronunciation.
- Instructors may want to use the audio library at the beginning of the class period to prepare students for the lecture or to review previously covered material. Other instructors like to use the audio library at the end of the class period to reinforce the material presented in class.
- Students can review terms at their own pace. This allows students to hear the terms whenever and how often they choose.
- Some instructors like to use the audio library for transcription exercises or spelling tests.
- As students become more familiar with the material, they can listen to the audio library and come to understand the medical terms as they are spoken. Sometimes students become very good at dividing medical terms into parts and defining them when they see the term, but in the real world, they often need to follow verbal directions and give verbal instructions. Being able to hear, understand, and use the term in everyday language is one of the goals of a veterinary medical terminology course.

Multimedia

A variety of multimedia resources (DVDs, videostreaming, computer-based presentations, etc.) help students visualize the topic of discussion and allow students to hear medical terms being used in context. Multimedia sources include pet food companies, veterinary clinics, state veterinary medical associations, the U.S. Department of Agriculture (USDA), veterinary schools, veterinary distributors, the Internet, and private vendors who produce client and educational style videos.

Case Studies

Case studies are a valuable resource because they clearly demonstrate the use of medical terms in a real setting. Additional case studies, for use in the classroom or as homework activities, are available in this Instructor's Manual.

Another form of the case study is to provide students with a list of 10 terms (which you choose so that the terms correlate). Students are then asked to make up their own case studies. At first, students often say that they do not have enough medical knowledge to complete this activity. However, most students come up with fairly accurate cases. If they do make up a case study that is inaccurate, it serves as a good topic for classroom discussion. As time progresses, students become very skilled at preparing case histories, know what information is helpful in taking case histories, and integrate information learned in other courses to make up more accurate case studies. Students seem to enjoy this activity as well.

Case study organization, for you and for students, should be based on the following:

- Signalment
- History and physical examination
- Laboratory reports
- Case summaries
- Consultation reports
- Surgical reports
- Discharge summaries

Suggestions for using case studies include:

- Holding stimulating class discussion.
- Providing spelling practice.
- Teaching different history-taking or reporting styles.
- Translating medical terminology into lay terms for clients (client education sheets).
- Encouraging students to research veterinary medical topics about diseases, conditions, or techniques.
- Learning abbreviations. (Instead of memorizing long lists of abbreviations, students learn them in context and by body system.)
- Expanding students' awareness of complex medical terms or medical terms that may not have been covered in class. (Providing pathology reports is an excellent way of demonstrating to students that they may not know all of the medical terms, but they can make sense of most of them.)
- Learning laboratory tests.
- Learning about medications and medication forms.

Crossword Puzzles

Medical terminology crossword puzzles and similar word searches are excellent ways to get students to interact with the material they are learning.

Crossword puzzles can be duplicated and provided to students to solve individually, or transparencies of the puzzles can be used as classroom activities. Crossword puzzle software can be purchased at many computer stores. Answer keys to the puzzles can be provided on the reverse side of the sheets given to students or duplicated and given to students after they work the puzzles.

Current Veterinary Medical Information Portfolio

A portfolio containing current veterinary medical articles is a useful resource. Articles from veterinary technician journals, breeder newsletters, and the Internet, or client education sheets can be laminated or stored in protective sheets in a three-ring binder. Students may choose articles from the portfolio to test their knowledge of medical terminology, to use in preparing reports, or to use when preparing class presentations. Students also may collect articles to add to the portfolio.

Suggestions for maintaining the portfolio include the following:

- Encourage students to make copies of the articles they like so that they can add them to their notes.
- Make sure the articles show the source and date of publication.
- Retire older articles and replace them with newer articles or compare the information in older articles with more current information.
- Make the portfolio available to all students.
- Allow students to use the articles to prepare reports. Also use the articles to spike interest about a topic in which many different medical terms are used and to stimulate classroom discussion to evaluate the accuracy of the information.

Reading Veterinary-Related Books to Arouse Student Interest

Assigning a veterinary-related book for students to read is one way to stimulate their interest in learning veterinary medical terminology. One suggestion is to have students read *Every Living Thing* by James Herriot and complete medical terminology worksheets based on terms presented in the book.

Visual Aids

Overhead transparencies or computer-based presentations (such as Power Point) are visual teaching aids used to complement written material. When creating your own presentations, use the following guidelines:

- Make sure the type is large enough to be read at a distance (at least 12-point type).
- Use colored pens, colored highlighters, or colored duplications for clarification during class.

- Duplicate case studies to be used for classroom discussion.
- Complete word division exercises for classroom demonstration.
- Use presentations for testing.
- Include example test questions to show students the exam format or to review material.
- Include discussion questions to direct student studying.
- Give students a printed copy for notetaking. Some of the printed copies can be left incomplete for students to fill in during lecture. For example, you can use a diagram to demonstrate blood flow through the heart.

Wall Charts and Posters

Wall charts and posters are effective learning tools if the print and pictures are large enough. These aids can be obtained from veterinary clinics or veterinary distributors or purchased through various catalogs.

Bulletin Board

A bulletin board (whether it is wall-mounted or electronic) is an effective way to communicate with students and to remind them of what they have learned and what they will learn. Review questions, pictures, and outlines can be displayed on a bulletin board for students to check. This will help students think about a class after a lecture and remind them about the key concepts of a section.

Models

Anatomic models are effective tools to demonstrate what body parts look like and how processes occur in the body. Live models help in correlating a body part from a photo to a live animal. Sometimes it is helpful to see where the elbow is on a live animal versus a skeleton. Photocopies of these models or body systems should be provided to students as well so that they can take accurate notes at the same time.

Personal Experiences

Providing students with personal experiences that relate to the material being covered helps them relate the material they are learning to what they will need in the real world. It is also an effective way to integrate the material covered in other courses.

Guest speakers from the veterinary field and laboratory setting also help students recognize the importance of understanding and using veterinary medical terminology. Videotaping guest speakers results in a library of useful teaching tools and serves as a substitute in case guest speakers cancel at the last minute. Field trips help students observe medical terminology being used in a work setting. A field trip may serve as a reward at the end of the course.

Pairing of Information

Many medical terms sound alike or can be related to another term. Pairs help students distinguish the difference between terms and the importance of recognizing this difference.

Suggestions for pairing of terms include the following:

- Post word pairs or duplicate a sheet of word pairs at the beginning of the course. This helps students get in the habit of studying terms in this fashion.
- Add to the list as the course progresses. If students want to add a pair that does not seem to fit the pattern, take time to explain why the terms do not fit.
- Use the list for drills and classroom activities.
- Test from the list.

Resource Files

Having your own set of resource files allows you to organize your ideas and enrich the material that worked well and to cull the material that did not work so well. Ways to get started include the following:

- Create a file folder for each major topic or textbook chapter.
- Arrange files in alphabetical order and allow space for expansion.
- As you come across information on a topic, add it to the file.
- Encourage students to add relevant material to the file. Students have a fresh outlook on what does and does not work, so use them as a resource.
- Include client education sheets and area newsletters, as they are useful sources of information. Class discussions can center around both correct and incorrect material.
- Add Internet information, both correct and incorrect, to your file. Remember that websites that end in .net are from major Internet providers, .com sites are businesses and can be added by anyone, .org sites are organizations (both nonprofit and service groups) and are considered more accurate than .com sources, .edu sites are from educational institutions, .gov sites are from government agencies, and .mil sites are from military facilities.
- Include veterinary medical newsletters published by area referral clinics or veterinary medical teaching hospitals. These newsletters serve as excellent sources of information. Consult area veterinarians for information about various schools.

Researching Topics

Having students prepare reports is a valuable teaching tool because it gives them experience seeking out and analyzing information. Reports can help students understand a topic, as well as the medical terminology used in the report.

Suggestions for the use of reports include the following:

- Assign students a medical topic that interests them.
- Have students make a copy of the article and submit it with their report.
- Have students study the article and be prepared to present it to the class.
- Assign the report well in advance so that students have enough time to find an article that interests them. You may find it necessary to provide students with various "stepping stones" for completing the final project; that is, this week they turn in their topics, next week they turn in their searches, the following week they provide an abstract, etc. This may help eliminate duplication of topics.
- Make sure each student uses a different article.
- Consider assigning specific articles from your resource file.
- If the article is written in lay terms, have students circle those terms and substitute the appropriate medical term.
- If the article is written in medical terms, have students circle those terms and substitute lay terms or definitions.
- Have students present their reports in oral or written form (may vary throughout the course).

Reading

Reading books on animal-related subjects is a good way for students to understand the importance of learning medical terminology. Students will have many opportunities to read textbooks and content-laden books on academic material throughout their courses. Another way to introduce them to medical terminology in everyday use is to have them read popular press books related to veterinary medicine. For example, you may assign weekly chapters for students to read and have them turn in three sets of answers to instructor-generated questions at three specified times during the course. This way students see how terms they are learning are used in a less structured way. It also teaches them concepts about veterinary medicine that would not get covered in a typical terminology course. Students should answer the questions in a general sense, using a dictionary if needed. The way the term is presented in the chapters is helpful in seeing how it is used, but should not replace dividing the word and defining each word part or using a dictionary. Sometimes students relate the term only to the chapter and answer the question only for the species involved in the chapter. Warn students of this.

PART III

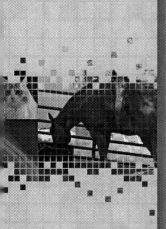

[Answers to Text Review Exercises]

Answers are shown in **boldface** type.

Chapter 1

Multiple Choice

1. **b**	11. **a**
2. **b**	12. **c**
3. **c**	13. **b**
4. **d**	14. **c**
5. **b**	15. **b**
6. **a**	16. **d**
7. **d**	17. **d**
8. **d**	18. **d**
9. **c**	19. **c**
10. **a**	20. **c**

Matching

1. **i**	8. **d**
2. **j**	9. **m**
3. **k**	10. **h**
4. **a**	11. **g**
5. **b**	12. **e**
6. **c**	13. **f**
7. **l**	

Fill in the Blanks

1. **gastric**
2. **hepatitis**
3. **osteomalacia**
4. **arthrodynia or arthralgia**
5. **endoscopy**

6. **cardiomegaly**
7. **renal**
8. **hemorrhage**
9. **gastropexy**
10. **chemotherapy**

Spell Check

1. **mucus**
2. **cystocentesis; urinalysis**
3. **diarrhea**
4. **cutaneous**
5. **anesthetic**

Word Part Identification

word root(s)

1. **hepat**/itis
2. **gastr**/o/**intestin**/al
3. **cardi**/o/logy
4. intra/**ven**/ous
5. **nephr**/osis

suffix

6. hepat/**itis**
7. gastr/o/intestin/**al**
8. cardi/o/**logy**
9. intra/ven/**ous**
10. nephr/**osis**

prefix

11. **hyper**/secretion
12. **peri**/card/itis
13. **endo**/cardi/um
14. **poly**/uria
15. ur/o/lith (*Urolith* does not contain a prefix.)

Crossword Puzzles

Prefix Puzzle

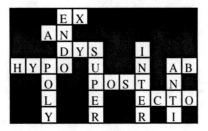

Suffix Puzzle

```
              R R H A G E
        G     R
      G R A P H Y
      A     E       P
      M A L A C I A     U
    C           T O M Y
    E     P   I   H
    N   E C T O M Y
    T     X   I       L
    E     Y   S T O M Y
    S           S     S
    I           I     I
    S C L E R O S I S
```

Medical Terms Puzzles

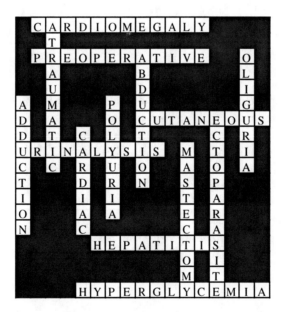

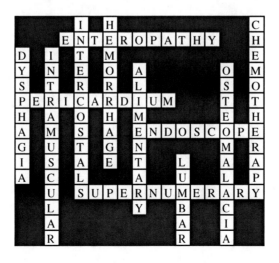

Word Search

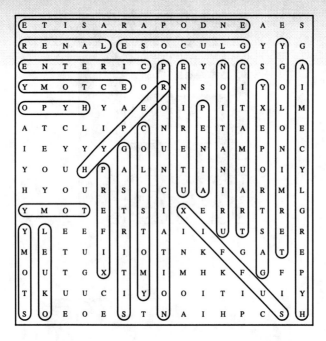

Case Study

A 5-year-old male neutered cat is presented to a veterinary clinic with **dysuria** (painful urination) and **oliguria** (scant urine production). Upon examination, the abdomen is <u>palpated</u> and **cystomegaly** (enlarged urinary bladder) is noted. After completing the examination, the veterinarian suspects an <u>obstruction</u> of the **urethra** (tube that carries urine from the urinary bladder to outside the body). Blood is taken for analysis, and the cat is admitted to the clinic. The cat is anesthetized and a urinary <u>catheter</u> is passed. Urine is collected for **urinalysis** (breakdown of urine into its components). In addition to the obstruction, the cat is treated for **cystitis** (inflammation of the urinary bladder).

1. palpated	**examined by feeling**
2. obstruction	**complete stoppage or impairment to passage**
3. catheter	**tube that is inserted into a body cavity to inject or remove fluid**

CHAPTER 2

Multiple Choice

1. **c**	11. **a**
2. **b**	12. **c**
3. **d**	13. **b**
4. **a**	14. **d**
5. **b**	15. **b**
6. **b**	16. **d**
7. **c**	17. **c**
8. **c**	18. **a**
9. **b**	19. **b**
10. **d**	20. **c**

Matching

1. **b, f**   6. **k**
2. **e**   7. **a**
3. **c**   8. **h**
4. **i, j**   9. **l**
5. **g, n**   10. **d, m**

Matching

11. **b**
12. **e**
13. **a**
14. **c**
15. **d**

Fill in the Blanks

1. **umbilicus**   14. **benign**
2. **Endocrine**   15. **hyster/o, metr/o, metr/i, metri/o,** and **uter/o**
3. **neoplasm**   16. **midsaggital**
4. **anomaly**   17. **transverse**
5. **thoracic**   18. **anatomy**
6. **palmar**   19. **physiology**
7. **cranial**   20. **lingual surface**
8. **cell**   21. **buccal surface**
9. **caudal** (or **inferior**) 22. **adduction**
10. **Hyperflexion**   23. **abduction**
11. **inguinal area**   24. **glands**
12. **mesentery**   25. **organ**
13. **-plasm**

Crossword Puzzle—Directional Terms and Planes of the Body

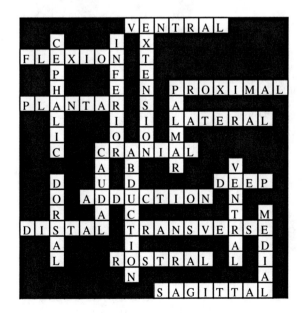

Crossword Puzzle—Organ Combining Forms

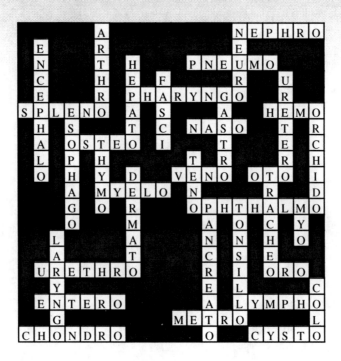

Diagrams

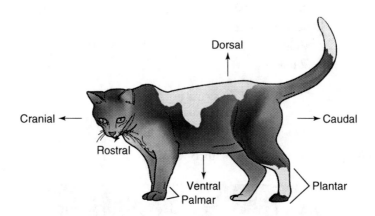

Figure 2–16 (cat)

A. **cranial**

B. **palmar**

C. **ventral**

D. **plantar**

E. **caudal**

F. **dorsal**

G. **rostral**

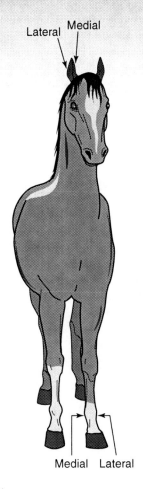

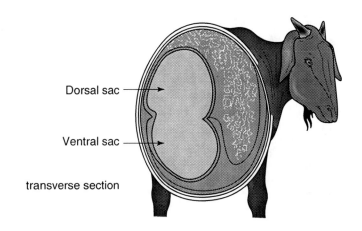

Figure 2–17 (horse)

A. **medial**
B. **lateral**
C. **medial**
D. **lateral**

Figure 2–18 (goat)

A. **dorsal sac**
B. **ventral sac**

The goat is sectioned through the transverse plane.

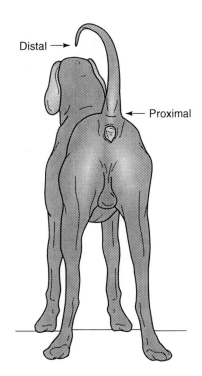

Figure 2–19 (dog)

A. **distal**
B. **proximal**

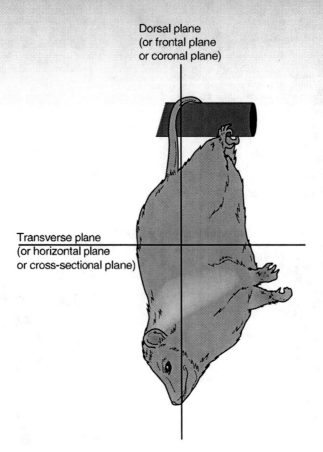

Figure 2–20 (opossum)

A. **transverse plane** (or **horizontal plane** or **cross-sectional plane**)
B. **dorsal plane** (or **frontal plane** or **coronal plane**)

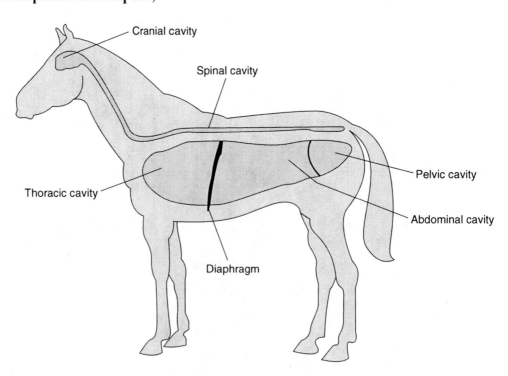

Figure 2–21 (horse)

A. **cranial cavity**
B. **spinal cavity**
C. **thoracic cavity**
D. **abdominal cavity**
E. **pelvic cavity**

Case Study

1. thoracic	**chest**
2. tumor	**mass of tissue**
3. cranial	**toward the head (crani/o means skull)**
4. hypertrophy	**increase in size (hyper means to increase; trophy means formation, development, and increase in size)**
5. malignant	**to spread and be life threatening**

CHAPTER 3

Multiple Choice

1. **c**	11. **b**	21. **a**
2. **b**	12. **d**	22. **d**
3. **a**	13. **b**	23. **b**
4. **d**	14. **c**	24. **c**
5. **c**	15. **b**	25. **b**
6. **d**	16. **a**	26. **c**
7. **b**	17. **b**	27. **c**
8. **b**	18. **c**	28. **c**
9. **a**	19. **c**	29. **d**
10. **b**	20. **d**	30. **a**

Matching

1. **e**	8. **k**
2. **d**	9. **a**
3. **c**	10. **m**
4. **b**	11. **g**
5. **i**	12. **f**
6. **h**	13. **l**
7. **j**	14. **n**

Matching

15. **b**	21. **a**
16. **d**	22. **e**
17. **d**	23. **a**
18. **a**	24. **d**
19. **c**	25. **g**
20. **f**	

Fill in the Blanks

1. **Dislocation; luxation**	11. **Chondromalacia**
2. **periosteum**	12. **extensor**
3. **meniscus**	13. **hyperextension**
4. **joints; articulations**	14. **adhesion**
5. **xiphoid process**	15. **brachycephalic**
6. **amputation**	16. **smooth, nonstriated (unstriated), visceral**
7. **sequestrum**	17. **onychectomy**
8. **varus**	18. **open or compound fracture**
9. **arthroscopy**	19. **linea alba**
10. **Ankylosis**	20. **muscle insertion**

21. **tendinitis**
22. **flexion**
23. **relaxation**
24. **depressor**
25. **superior**
26. **transverse**
27. **oblique**
28. **crepitation**
29. **comminuted fractures**
30. **hip dysplasia**

True or False

1. **True**
2. **False**
3. **False**
4. **True**
5. **True**

Crossword Puzzle

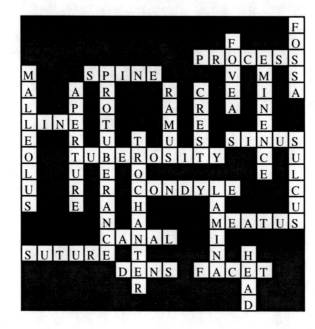

Word Search

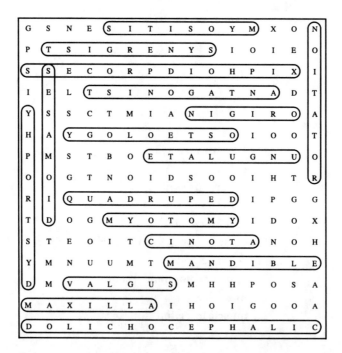

Diagrams

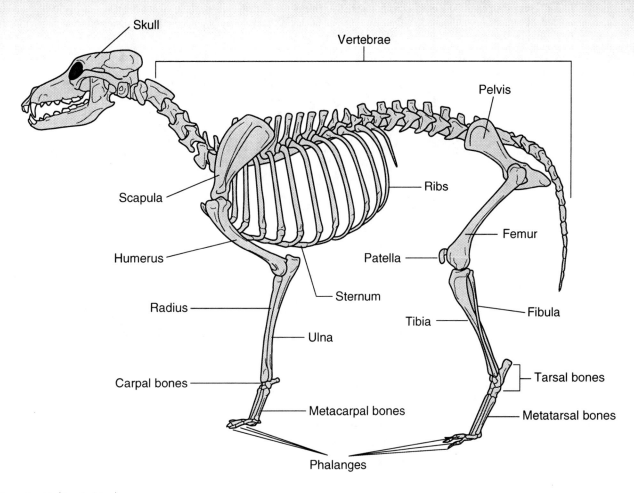

Skull

Vertebrae

Pelvis

Scapula

Ribs

Femur

Humerus

Patella

Sternum

Radius

Fibula

Tibia

Ulna

Carpal bones

Tarsal bones

Metacarpal bones

Metatarsal bones

Phalanges

Figure 3–31 (dog skeleton)

A. **skull**
B. **vertebrae**
C. **pelvis**
D. **scapula**
E. **humerus**
F. **radius**
G. **carpal bones**
H. **ribs**
I. **patella**
J. **tibia**
K. **sternum**
L. **ulna**
M. **metacarpal bones**
N. **phalanges**
O. **femur**
P. **fibula**
Q. **tarsal bones**
R. **metatarsal bones**

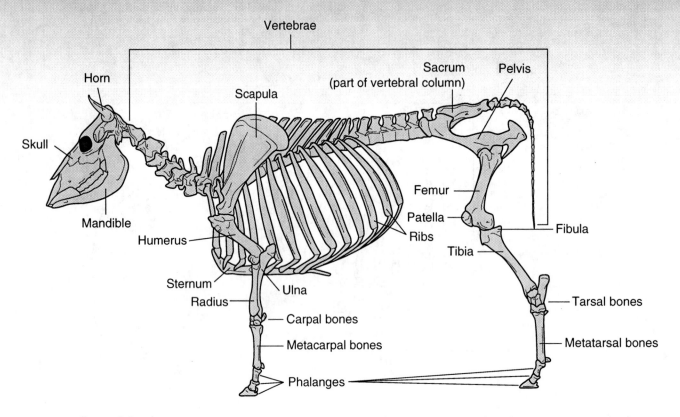

Figure 3–32 (bovine skeleton)

A. **skull**
B. **horn**
C. **vertebrae**
D. **scapula**
E. **sacrum (part of vertebral column)**
F. **pelvis**
G. **mandible**
H. **humerus**
I. **sternum**
J. **radius**
K. **ulna**

L. **carpal bones**
M. **metacarpal bones**
N. **phalanges**
O. **femur**
P. **patella**
Q. **ribs**
R. **tibia**
S. **fibula**
T. **tarsal bones**
U. **metatarsal bones**

CHAPTER 4

Multiple Choice

1. **a**	11. **b**
2. **d**	12. **a**
3. **b**	13. **c**
4. **c**	14. **d**
5. **b**	15. **d**
6. **c**	16. **c**
7. **b**	17. **b**
8. **a**	18. **a**
9. **c**	19. **c**
10. **b**	20. **d**

Matching

1. **d**	6. **i**
2. **f**	7. **j**
3. **a**	8. **c**
4. **g**	9. **e**
5. **h**	10. **b**

Crossword Puzzle

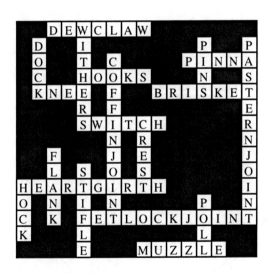

Dog and Cat Word Search

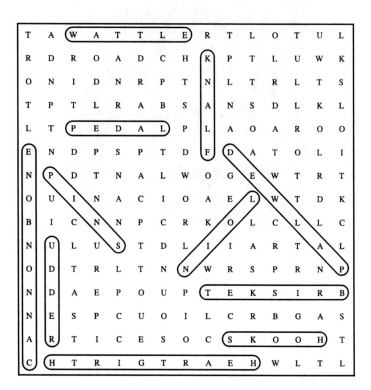

Ruminant Word Search

Equine Word Search

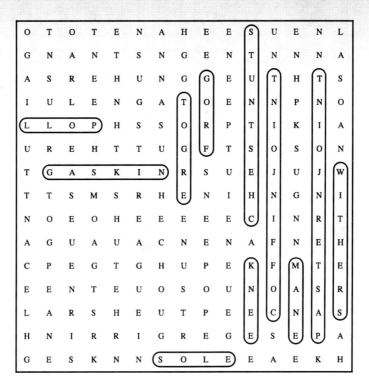

Swine Word Search

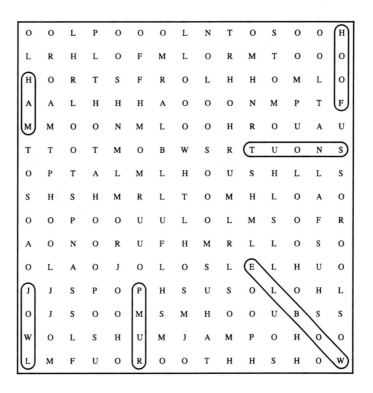

Diagrams

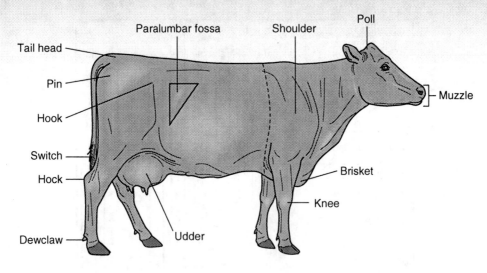

Figure 4–10 (cow)

A. **tail head**

B. **pin**

C. **hook**

D. **switch**

E. **hock**

F. **dewclaw**

G. **shoulder**

H. **poll**

I. **muzzle**

J. **brisket**

K. **knee**

L. **udder**

M. **paralumbar fossa**

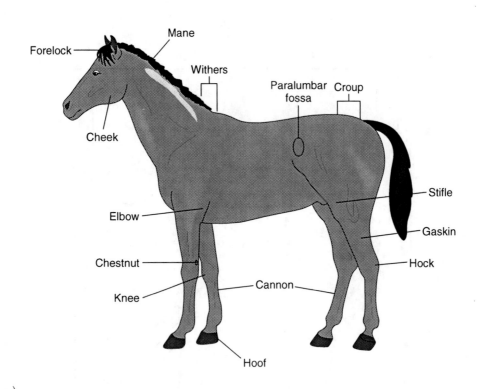

Figure 4–11 (horse)

A. **forelock**

B. **cheek**

C. **mane**

D. **withers**

E. **elbow**

F. **chestnut**

G. **hoof**

H. **croup**

I. **stifle**

J. **gaskin**

K. **hock**

L. **knee**

M. **cannon**

N. **paralumbar fossa**

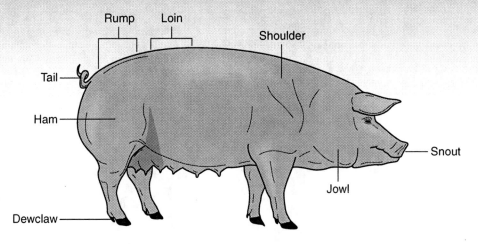

Figure 4–12 (swine)

A. **tail**
B. **rump**
C. **loin**
D. **shoulder**

E. **snout**
F. **jowl**
G. **dewclaw**
H. **ham**

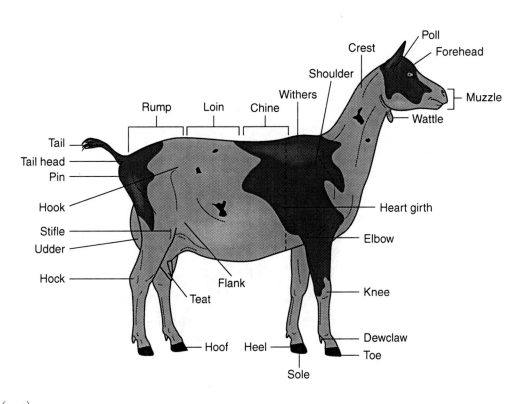

Figure 4–13 (goat)

A. **tail**
B. **tail head**
C. **pin**
D. **hook**
E. **stifle**
F. **udder**
G. **hock**
H. **teat**
I. **flank**

J. **hoof**
K. **heel**
L. **sole**
M. **toe**
N. **dewclaw**
O. **knee**
P. **elbow**
Q. **heart girth**
R. **wattle**

S. **muzzle**
T. **forehead**
U. **poll**
V. **crest**
W. **shoulder**
X. **withers**
Y. **chine**
Z. **loin**
AA. **rump**

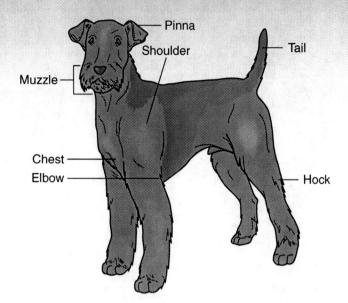

Figure 4–14 (dog)

A. **muzzle**

B. **chest**

C. **elbow**

D. **pinna**

E. **shoulder**

F. **tail**

G. **hock**

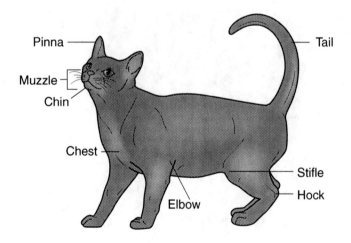

Figure 4–15 (cat)

A. **pinna**

B. **muzzle**

C. **chin**

D. **chest**

E. **elbow**

F. **hock**

G. **stifle**

H. **tail**

Labeling

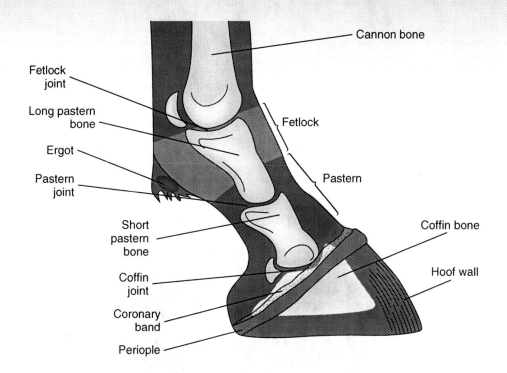

CHAPTER 5

Multiple Choice

1. **c**	11. **c**
2. **b**	12. **c**
3. **d**	13. **d**
4. **d**	14. **c**
5. **b**	15. **b**
6. **a**	16. **d**
7. **c**	17. **b**
8. **b**	18. **d**
9. **b**	19. **d**
10. **c**	20. **a**

Matching

1. **b**	7. **f**
2. **d**	8. **i**
3. **g**	9. **c**
4. **h**	10. **c**
5. **i**	11. **e**
6. **a**	

Matching

12. **d**	17. **c**
13. **f**	18. **h**
14. **e**	19. **j**
15. **i**	20. **a**
16. **g**	21. **b**

Fill in the Blanks

1. **whelp; pup**
2. **kitten**
3. **foal**
4. **calf**
5. **kid**
6. **lamb**
7. **pig; shoat (not used much anymore)**
8. **kits**
9. **pups**
10. **cria**

11. **herd**
12. **herd**
13. **flock**
14. **flock**
15. **herd**
16. **hatchling**
17. **chick**
18. **fawn**
19. **capon**
20. **clutch**

Crossword Puzzle

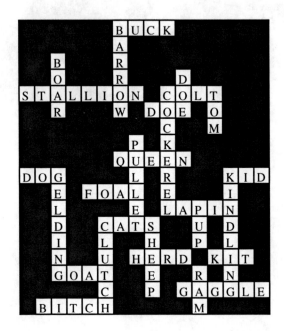

CHAPTER 6

Multiple Choice

1. **c**
2. **a**
3. **d**
4. **c**
5. **b**
6. **a**
7. **c**
8. **c**
9. **d**
10. **a**

11. **b**
12. **b**
13. **c**
14. **a**
15. **a**
16. **d**
17. **b**
18. **d**
19. **c**
20. **b**

Matching

1. **c**
2. **d**
3. **f**
4. **e**
5. **h**

6. **g**
7. **j**
8. **i**
9. **b**
10. **a**

Fill in the Blanks

1. **tongue**
2. **mouth**
3. **lips**
4. **abdomen**
5. **teeth**

Spelling

1. vulvulus **volvulus** volvolus
2. achalsia **achalasia** achaelasia
3. jaundise jawndise **jaundice**
4. eviserate **eviscerate** eviscerate
5. **ascites** asites ascetes

Crossword Puzzle—Disease Terms

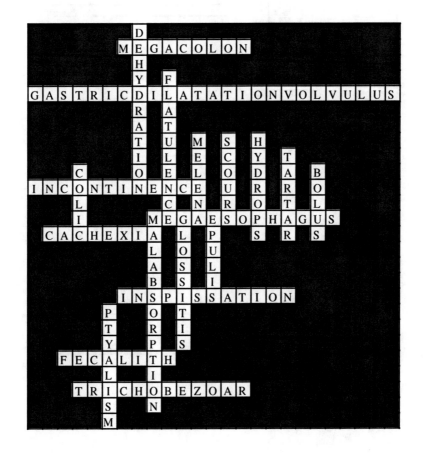

Crossword Puzzle—Digestive Organs

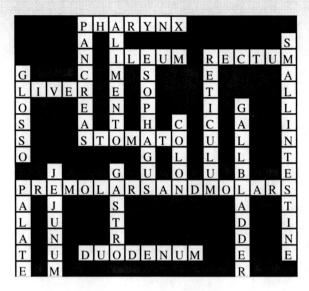

Word Search

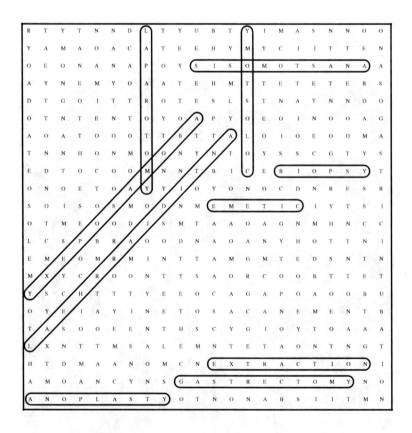

anastomosis	anoplasty
laparotomy	colostomy
gastrectomy	abomasopexy
emetic	biopsy
extraction	antidiarrheal

Diagrams

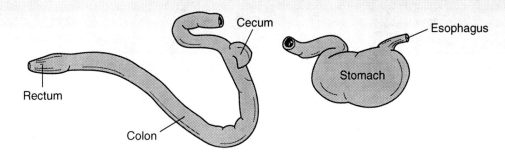

(A) **Dog**

Figure 6–40: part (a) dog

A. **rectum**
B. **colon**
C. **stomach**
D. **esophagus**
E. **cecum**

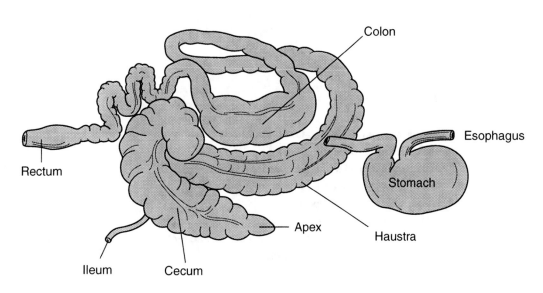

(B) **Horse**

Figure 6–40: part (b) horse

A. **rectum**   E. **haustra**
B. **ileum**   F. **stomach**
C. **cecum**   G. **esophagus**
D. **apex**   H. **colon**

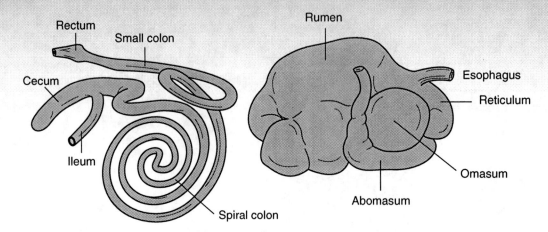

(C) **Ruminant**

Figure 6–40: part (c) ruminant

A. **ileum**   F. **reticulum**

B. **spiral colon**   G. **esophagus**

C. **cecum**   H. **rumen**

D. **abomasum**   I. **small colon**

E. **omasum**   J. **rectum**

Case Studies

1.	yr	**year**
2.	F/S	**female/spayed**
3.	hx	**history**
4.	quidding	**condition in which food is taken into the mouth and chewed but falls from the mouth**
5.	ptyalism	**excessive salivation**
6.	prehending	**grasping food/collecting food into the oral cavity**
7.	incisors	**front teeth used for cutting**
8.	malocclusion	**abnormal contact between teeth**
9.	dental arcades	**arches in which teeth are arranged**
10.	premolars	**cheek teeth found between the canine teeth and molars**
11.	molars	**most caudally located permanent cheek teeth**
12.	extraction	**removal/surgical removal of a tooth**
13.	anesthesia	**without sensation or feeling**
14.	analgesics	**substances that relieve pain without affecting consciousness**
15.	postoperatively	**after surgery**
16.	wk	**week**
17.	acute	**rapidly occurring**
18.	emesis	**vomiting**
19.	hemorrhagic	**pertaining to bursting forth of blood/bleeding**
20.	diarrhea	**abnormal frequency and liquidity of fecal material**
21.	lethargy	**condition of drowsiness or indifference**
22.	anorexia	**lack of appetite**
23.	pyrexic	**feverish**
24.	dehydrated	**condition of excessive loss of body water or fluid**
25.	auscultated	**listened to (with an instrument)**
26.	stool	**feces**
27.	lymphopenia	**decreased number of lymphocytes**

28. dx	**diagnosis**
29. canine	**dog or member of the dog family**
30. enteritis	**inflammation of the small intestines**
31. IV	**intravenous**
32. secondary	**not the primary cause**
33. septicemia	**blood condition in which pathogenic microorganisms or their toxins are present**
34. expired	**died**
35. necropsy	**examination of an animal body after death**
36. intestinal villi	**tiny hairlike projections on the small intestinal wall**
37. crypt	**blind sac**
38. disinfected	**killed or inhibited the growth of microorganisms on inanimate objects**

CHAPTER 7

Multiple Choice

1. **b**	8. **b**	15. **a**
2. **c**	9. **c**	16. **d**
3. **d**	10. **d**	17. **b**
4. **b**	11. **d**	18. **a**
5. **a**	12. **b**	19. **d**
6. **c**	13. **c**	20. **b**
7. **a**	14. **b**	

Matching

1. **h**	11. **g**
2. **i**	12. **j**
3. **d**	13. **o**
4. **k**	14. **b**
5. **a**	15. **f**
6. **c**	16. **s**
7. **l**	17. **q**
8. **e**	18. **p**
9. **n**	19. **t**
10. **m**	20. **r**

Fill in the Blanks

1. **urine** or **pertaining to urinary organs**
2. **kidney**
3. **glucose in the urine**
4. **urinary bladder stone**
5. **elimination of a substance**

Spelling

1. urinanalysis **urinalysis** urinealisis
2. **nephron** nefron nephrone
3. homostasis **homeostasis** homeostatis
4. **polydipsia** polydypsia polydyspsia
5. calkulus kalkulus **calculus**

Crossword Puzzles

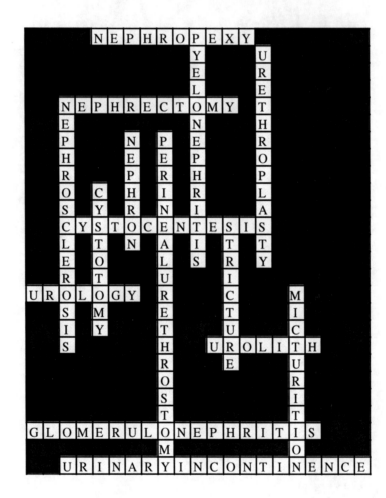

Diagram

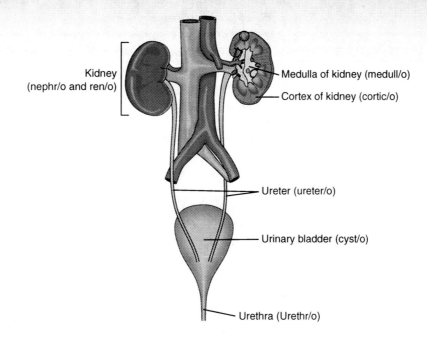

Figure 7–14

A. **kidney (nephr/o** and **ren/o)**
B. **ureter (ureter/o)**
C. **urinary bladder (cyst/o)**
D. **urethra (urethr/o)**
E. **medulla of kidney (medull/o)**
F. **cortex of kidney (cortic/o)**

Case Studies

1.	year	**yr**
2.	male neutered	**M/N**
3.	difficulty urinating	**dysuria**
4.	blood in the urine	**hematuria**
5.	examination of urine by breaking it into its components	**urinalysis**
6.	inserting a needle in the urinary bladder and withdrawing urine	**cystocentesis**
7.	erythrocytes	**RBCs, or red blood cells**
8.	inflammation of the urinary bladder	**cystitis**
9.	X-ray	**radiograph**
10.	urinary bladder stones	**urolith, cystolith, or urinary stone calculus**
11.	incision into the urinary bladder	**cystotomy**
12.	M/N	**male/neutered**
13.	DLH	**domestic long hair**
14.	inappropriately urinating	**eliminating urine either at the wrong time or in the wrong place**
15.	dehydrated	**condition of excessive loss of body water or fluid**
16.	auscultated	**listened to (with an instrument)**
17.	cystomegaly	**urinary bladder enlargement**
18.	urethra	**singular tube extending from the urinary bladder to the outside of the body**
19.	urinate	**act of voiding urine**

20.	dx'd	diagnosed
21.	urethral obstruction	blockage of the urethra so that urine flow out of the body is compromised
22.	anesthetized	produced lack of sensation
23.	inhalant anesthesia	gas form of drug that produces lack of sensation
24.	urinary catheter	hollow tube that is inserted through the urethra into the urinary bladder (usually to collect urine, but may be to inject contrast material or air)
25.	perineum	region between the scrotum/vulva and anus
26.	IV	intravenous
27.	UA	urinalysis
28.	pH	hydrogen ion concentration that in urine dictates acidity or alkalinity
29.	leukocytes	white blood cells
30.	specific gravity	measurement that reflects the amount of wastes, minerals, and solids in urine
31.	struvite crystals	type of angular solid (crystal) that is comprised of magnesium ammonium phosphate hexahydrate
32.	cystitis	inflammation of the urinary bladder
33.	cow	intact female bovine that has given birth
34.	off feed	not eating; anorexic
35.	polyuric	increased urination
36.	hematuria	blood in the urine
37.	rectal palpation	to examine by palpation by inserting gloved arm into the animal's rectum
38.	nephromegaly	kidney enlargement
39.	diagnosis	determination of the cause of disease
40.	pyelonephritis	inflammation of the renal pelvis and kidney
41.	UA	urinalysis
42.	culture and sensitivity	test in which sample is collected and streaked on agar in order to grow any bacteria present; sensitivity tests involve antibiotic-laden discs to determine to which antibiotics the cultured bacteria are sensitive (or which antibiotic is effective)

CHAPTER 8

Multiple Choice

1.	c	11.	b
2.	b	12.	c
3.	a	13.	b
4.	d	14.	d
5.	c	15.	b
6.	b	16.	c
7.	c	17.	d
8.	d	18.	a
9.	d	19.	b
10.	d	20.	d

Matching

1.	d	6.	j
2.	f	7.	b
3.	g	8.	a
4.	i	9.	c
5.	h	10.	e

Fill in the Blanks

1. **vessel**
2. **vein**
3. **valve**
4. **heart**
5. **all**

Trace the flow of blood through the heart.

6. **cranial vena cava; caudal vena cava; right atrium**
7. **right atrioventricular (or right AV) valve; tricuspid valve**
8. **pulmonary valve or pulmonary semilunar valve; pulmonary artery**
9. **pulmonary vein**
10. **left atrioventicular (or left AV) valve; mitral valve; left ventricle**
11. **aortic valve or aortic semilunar valve**

Spelling

1. cianosis cyianosis **cyanosis**
2. hypokapnea **hypocapnia** hypocapnea
3. vasodialation **vasodilation** vasodilatation
4. **diastole** diastoly diastooly
5. **systole** sistolle sistole

Crossword Puzzle

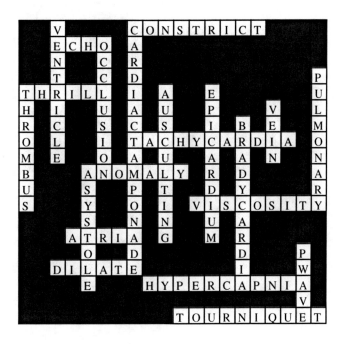

Diagrams

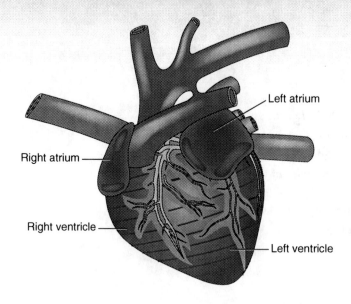

Figure 8–23

A. **right atrium**
B. **right ventricle**
C. **left atrium**
D. **left ventricle**

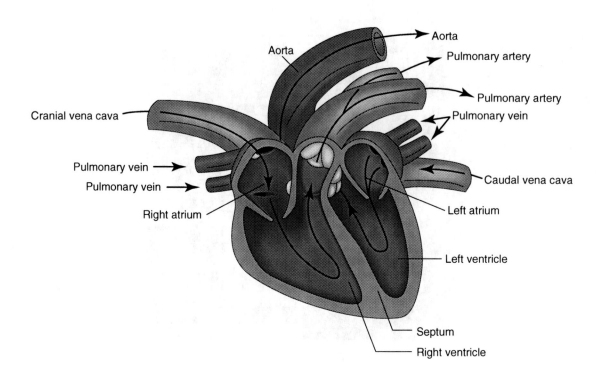

Figure 8–24

A. **cranial vena cava**
B. **aorta**
C. **pulmonary artery**
D. **pulmonary artery**
E. **pulmonary vein**

F. **pulmonary vein**
G. **left atrium**
H. **left ventricle**
I. **septum**
J. **right ventricle**

K. **aorta (to arteries of the body)**
L. **caudal vena cava**
M. **right atrium**
N. **pulmonary vein**
O. **pulmonary vein**

Case Studies

1.	lethargy	**condition of drowsiness or indifference**
2.	syncope	**temporary suspension of respiration and circulation**
3.	cyanotic	**bluish tinge to skin and mucous membranes**
4.	cardiac arrhythmia	**abnormal heart rhythm**
5.	tachycardia	**abnormally rapid heart rate**
6.	ECG	**electrocardiogram**
7.	radiograph	**record of ionizing radiation used to visualize internal body structures; also called X-ray**
8.	cardiomegaly	**heart enlargement**
9.	diagnosis	**determination of the cause of disease**
10.	cardiomyopathy	**disease of heart muscle**
11.	off feed	**not eating; anorexic**
12.	PE	**physical examination**
13.	tachycardia	**abnormally rapid heart beat**
14.	tachypnea	**abnormally rapid breathing**
15.	dyspnea	**difficulty breathing**
16.	pyrexia	**feverish**
17.	thorax	**chest area**
18.	rumen	**largest compartment that serves as a fermentation vat of the ruminant's stomach**
19.	prophylactic	**prevention**
20.	acute	**having a rapid onset**
21.	traumatic	**pertaining to, resulting from, or causing injury**
22.	reticuloperitonitis	**inflammation of the peritoneal cavity due to its contamination by contents leaking from the reticulum**
23.	acute traumatic reticuloperitonitis	**acute disease of ruminants seen when swallowed metallic objects fall into the reticulum of the ruminant stomach, pierce the reticulum wall, and cause contamination in the peritoneal cavity (commonly called hardware disease)**
24.	reticulum	**most cranial compartment of the ruminant; the forestomach**
25.	ruminant	**cud-chewing animal that has a forestomach, which allows for fermentation of ingesta**
26.	peritoneal cavity	**space in the abdominal cavity between the parietal and visceral peritoneum**
27.	diaphragm	**muscle separating the chest and abdomen**
28.	pericardial sac	**space between the membrane surrounding the heart (pericardium) and the heart itself**
29.	pericarditis	**inflammation of the pericardium**
30.	balling gun	**tool used to administer pills or magnets to livestock**

CHAPTER 9

Multiple Choice

1.	**c**	11.	**b**
2.	**d**	12.	**d**
3.	**b**	13.	**d**
4.	**d**	14.	**b**
5.	**a**	15.	**a**
6.	**a**	16.	**c**
7.	**c**	17.	**d**
8.	**d**	18.	**b**
9.	**a**	19.	**b**
10.	**b**	20.	**d**

Matching

1. **d**
2. **a**
3. **c**
4. **b**
5. **e**
6. **i**
7. **f**
8. **h**
9. **l**
10. **o**
11. **n**
12. **g**
13. **j**
14. **k**
15. **m**

Fill in the Blanks

1. **oxygen**
2. **nose**
3. **lung**
4. **lungs or air**
5. **the process of bringing in fresh air**

Spelling

1. pnuemonia **pneumonia** pnuemohnia
2. asfyxiation asphixiation **asphyxiation**
3. mucous mukus **mucus**
4. astmah **asthma** asmah
5. diafragm diaphram **diaphragm**

Crossword Puzzle

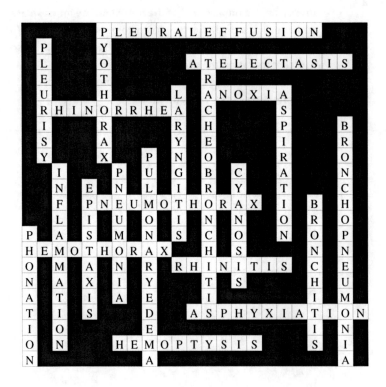

Diagram

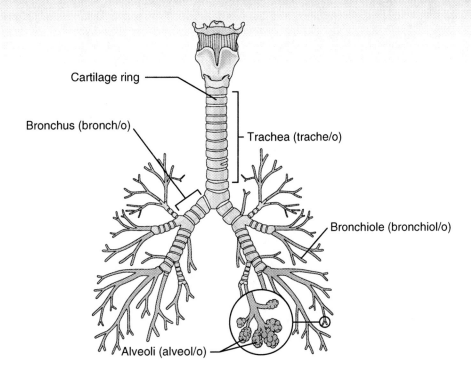

Figure 9–18

A. **cartilage ring**
B. **bronchus (bronch/o)**
C. **trachea (trache/o)**
D. **bronchiole (bronchiol/o)**
E. **alveoli (alveol/o)**

Case Studies

1.	endotracheal tube	**tube placed through the oral cavity, pharynx, and larynx into the windpipe**
2.	intubate	**to place an endotracheal tube**
3.	inspiratory dyspnea	**difficulty breathing when breathing in**
4.	cough	**sudden noisy expulsion of air from the lungs**
5.	cyanotic	**bluish tinge to the skin and mucous membranes**
6.	diagnosis	**determination of the cause of disease**
7.	laryngeal spasm	**sudden involuntary contractions or tightening of the voice box**
8.	tracheotomy	**incision into the windpipe**
9.	anorexia	**lack of appetite**
10.	pyrexic	**feverish**
11.	mucopurulent nasal discharge	**fluid from the nose and nasal cavity that contains pus and mucus**
12.	auscultation	**process of listening (with an instrument)**
13.	rales	**fine or coarse interrupted crackling noise coming from collapsed or fluid-filled alveoli during inspiration; also called crackles and crepitation**
14.	bovine	**biological name for cattle**
15.	pneumonic	**pertaining to the lungs or air**

CHAPTER 10

Multiple Choice

1. **c**
2. **b**
3. **d**
4. **c**
5. **c**
6. **b**
7. **b**
8. **d**
9. **a**
10. **c**
11. **b**
12. **c**
13. **b**
14. **d**
15. **c**
16. **b**
17. **c**
18. **d**
19. **b**
20. **a**

Matching

1. **d**
2. **f**
3. **i**
4. **l**
5. **p**
6. **b**
7. **m**
8. **e**
9. **c**
10. **k**
11. **g**
12. **j**
13. **n**
14. **h**
15. **a**
16. **o**
17. **u**
18. **w**
19. **r**
20. **x**
21. **s**
22. **z**
23. **v**
24. **q**
25. **t**
26. **y**

Fill in the Blanks

1. **skin**
2. **hair**
3. **middle layer of skin**
4. **deepest layer of skin**
5. **fluid-filled lesions**

Spelling

1. pruritis **pruritus** puritis
2. komedo **comedo** comedoe
3. **alopecia** ahlopesia alopecea
4. **hidrosis** hydrosis hihdrosis
5. manje mainge **mange**

Crossword Puzzle

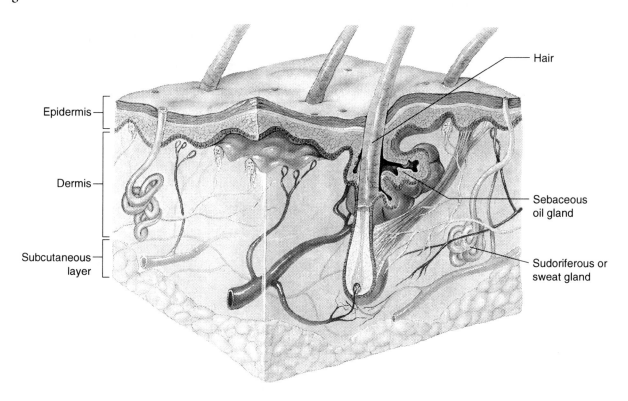

```
                        G                   L A C E R A T I O N
                        R                   D
          I N C I S I O N A L B I O P S Y
                        U       D                   P
                  P O L Y P     O                   I
                        O   P   C                   L
          Q U I C K     M   U   Y   H               O
                A   D       R   T   Y   P E T E C H I A
                U   I       P   E   O               E
          C Y S T   I       U       S   C E R U M E N
                E   F       R       E               T
  C           R   X F O L I A T I V E               I   K
  O           I   O       C   A                     O   E
  N           Z   C I R C U M S C R I B E D         N   R
  T           A   U       A   T                         A
  U           T   S       L   I                         T
  S           I   E       I   L                         O
  S H E D D I N G         Z   E                         S
  I           O           E           A B S C E S S     I
  O     H O R N     U N D E R C O A T                   S
  N                         I
              O N Y C H O M Y C O S I S
                            N
```

Diagram

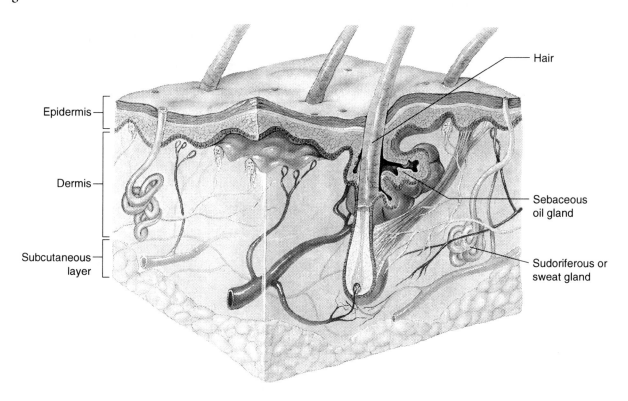

- Epidermis
- Dermis
- Subcutaneous layer
- Hair
- Sebaceous oil gland
- Sudoriferous or sweat gland

Figure 10–26

A. **hair**

B. **epidermis**

C. **dermis**

D. **subcutaneous layer**

E. **sudoriferous or sweat gland**

F. **sebaceous oil gland**

Case Studies

1. pruritus	**itchiness**
2. dermatitis	**inflammation of the skin**
3. otitis	**inflammation of the ear**
4. skin scrapes	**microscopic examination of the skin for the presence of mites; skin is sampled by taking a scalpel blade across an area of skin that is squeezed or raised so that the sample contains a deep skin sample**
5. dermatologist	**skin specialist**
6. atopy	**hypersensitivity reaction in animals involving pruritus with secondary dermatitis; also called allergies or allergic dermatitis**
7. intradermal skin testing	**injection of test substances into the skin layer to observe for a reaction**
8. hypoallergenic	**no or reduced potential to induce allergic reaction**
9. hyposensitization	**decreased response to an allergen (by injecting small amounts of an allergen into an animal and gradually increasing the amount of allergen present with each successive injection)**
10. pyoderma	**skin disease containing pus**
11. IM	**intramuscular**
12. ruminating	**process of bringing up food material from the stomach to the mouth for further chewing**
13. R	**right**
14. PE	**physical examination**
15. HR	**heart rate**
16. RR	**respiration rate**
17. palpation	**act of examining by feeling**
18. abscess	**localized collection of pus**
19. lancing	**to open or pierce with a lancet (scalpel blade) to allow drainage**
20. antiseptic	**chemical agent that kills or prevents the growth of microorganisms on living tissue**

CHAPTER 11

Multiple Choice

1. **b**	11. **d**
2. **d**	12. **c**
3. **c**	13. **c**
4. **a**	14. **d**
5. **c**	15. **b**
6. **b**	16. **c**
7. **c**	17. **b**
8. **d**	18. **a**
9. **c**	19. **a**
10. **b**	20. **b**

Matching

1. **h**	7. **d**	13. **p**
2. **a**	8. **e**	14. **q**
3. **b**	9. **m**	15. **r**
4. **c**	10. **o**	16. **j**
5. **f**	11. **l**	17. **i**
6. **g**	12. **k**	18. **n**

Fill in the Blanks

1. **thyroid gland**
2. **adrenal gland**
3. **having an affinity for**
4. **yellow**
5. **body**

Spelling

1. pancrease pancreus **pancrea**s
2. dyuretic diyuretic **diuretic**
3. pitwoitary **pituitary** pitootary
4. **hypothalamus** hypothalmus hypothalmis
5. gonids **gonads** goknads

Word Scramble

1. **anabolism**
2. **catabolism**
3. **hyperglycemia**
4. **pancreatitis**
5. **gonad**
6. **thyroidectomy**
7. **endocrinology**
8. **gluconeogenesis**
9. **synthetic**
10. **hypothyroidism**

Crossword Puzzle

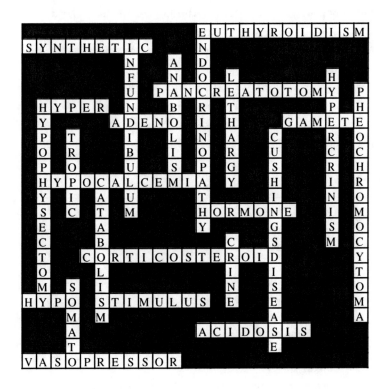

Diagram

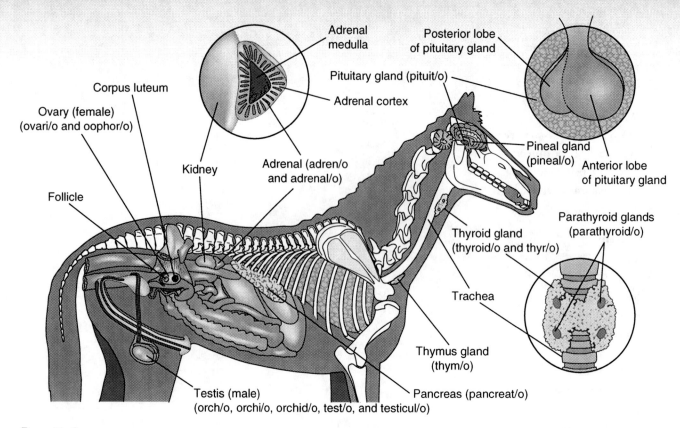

Figure 11–9

A. **follicle**

B. **ovary (female) (ovari/o and oophor/o)**

C. **corpus luteum**

D. **kidney**

E. **adrenal gland (adren/o and adrenal/o)**

F. **adrenal cortex**

G. **adrenal medulla**

H. **pituitary gland (pituit/o)**

I. **posterior lobe of pituitary gland**

J. **pineal gland (pineal/o)**

K. **anterior lobe of pituitary gland**

L. **parathyroid glands (parathyroid/o)**

M. **thyroid gland (thyroid/o and thyr/o)**

N. **trachea**

O. **thymus gland (thym/o)**

P. **pancreas (pancreat/o)**

Q. **testis (male) (orch/o, orchi/o, orchid/o, test/o, and testicul/o)**

Case Studies

1.	yr	**year**
2.	M/N	**male/neutered**
3.	T	**temperature**
4.	HR	**heart rate**
5.	BPM	**beats per minute**
6.	#	**pound(s) (when used after a number)**
7.	alopecia	**hair loss resulting in patches of baldness**
8.	lethargic	**condition of drowsiness or indifference**
9.	cm	**centimeter**
10.	lateral	**on the side**
11.	proximal	**nearest midline or nearest the beginning of a structure**
12.	elbow	**joint between the humerus and ulna/radius**
13.	medial	**toward midline**
14.	hock	**tarsus; joint between the tibia/fibula and metatarsal bones in the rear limb**

15. anesthetized	**provided lack of sensation**
16. BID	**twice daily**
17. d	**days**
18. hypothyroid	**less-than-normal levels of thyroid hormone**
19. yr	**year**
20. F/S	**female/spayed**
21. DSH	**domestic shorthair (cat)**
22. tachycardic	**abnormally rapid heart rate**
23. emaciated	**abnormally thin or wasted**
24. lethargic	**condition of drowsiness or indifference**
25. T	**temperature**
26. HR	**heart rate**
27. BPM	**beats per minute**
28. RR	**respiratory rate**
29. palpation	**act of examining by feeling**
30. vein	**vessel that carries blood toward the heart**
31. CBC	**complete blood count**
32. chem screen	**chemistry screen or series of tests run on serum to assess state of an organ; also called chem panel**
33. T_4	**thyroxine (one of the thyroid hormones)**
34. BUN	**blood urea nitrogen**
35. creatinine	**product of protein metabolism that is excreted through the kidney (becomes elevated with kidney disease)**
36. hypercholesterolemia	**abnormally high levels of cholesterol in the blood**
37. radioactive iodine treatments	**administration of radioactive iodine to suppress thyroid function; also called chemical thyroidectomy**
38. thyroidectomy	**surgical removal of the thyroid gland**

CHAPTER 12

Multiple Choice

1. **d**	8. **a**	15. **d**
2. **b**	9. **c**	16. **b**
3. **a**	10. **d**	17. **c**
4. **d**	11. **c**	18. **c**
5. **a**	12. **b**	19. **c**
6. **c**	13. **d**	20. **b**
7. **b**	14. **b**	

Matching

1. **d**	6. **f**
2. **h**	7. **e**
3. **j**	8. **a**
4. **g**	9. **c**
5. **i**	10. **b**

Fill in the Blanks

1. **vagina**
2. **uterus**
3. **penis**
4. **testis**
5. **spermatozoa**

Spelling

1. **cryptorchidism** criptorchidism cryptorchydism
2. mastis **mastitis** masitits
3. zigoat zygoat **zygote**
4. syesis **cyesis** ciesis
5. **neuter** nueter newter

Word Building

1. **py/o; metr/o; pyometra**
2. **par/a; ovari/o; parovarian**
3. **ur/o; genit/o; (-al); urogenital**
4. **lact/o; gen/o; (-ic); lactogenic**
5. **hysteri/o; -ectomy; hysterectomy**

Crossword Puzzle

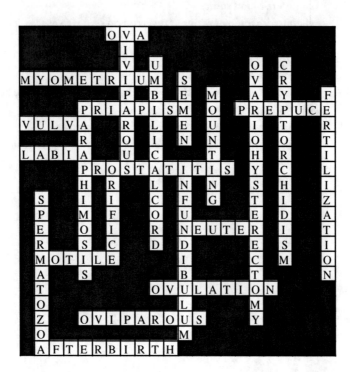

Case Studies

1.	yr	**year**
2.	F	**female**
3.	lethargy	**condition of drowsiness or indifference**
4.	anorexia	**lack of appetite**
5.	PU/PD	**polyuria/polydipsia; increased urination/increased drinking or thirst**
6.	bitch	**intact female dog**
7.	proestrus	**period of the estrous cycle before sexual receptivity**
8.	PE	**physical examination**
9.	pyrexic	**feverish**
10.	tachypneic	**abnormally rapid breathing**
11.	abdominal	**area between the thoracic and pelvic cavities**
12.	palpation	**act of examining by feeling**

13.	uterus	**thick-walled, hollow organ of females in which the fetus develops**
14.	purulent	**puslike**
15.	vaginal	**pertaining to the vagina**
16.	CBC	**complete blood count**
17.	chem panel	**chemistry screen or series of tests run on serum to assess state of an organ; also called chem screen**
18.	leukocytosis	**abnormally high number of white blood cells**
19.	dx	**diagnosis**
20.	pyometra	**pus in the uterus**
21.	OHE	**ovariohysterectomy**
22.	yr	**year**
23.	intact	**not sexually altered**
24.	M	**male**
25.	stranguria	**slow or painful urination**
26.	hematuria	**blood in the urine**
27.	PE	**physical examination**
28.	pyrexia	**feverish**
29.	anorexia	**lack of appetite**
30.	gait	**the way an animal moves**
31.	rectal palpation	**act of examining by inserting a gloved arm into the animal's rectum**
32.	prostate gland	**gland that secretes a thick fluid that aids in motility of sperm surrounding the urethra**
33.	bilaterally	**both sides**
34.	hx	**history**
35.	recurrent	**occurring again**
36.	UTI	**urinary tract infection**
37.	radiographs	**records of ionizing radiation used to visualize internal body structures; also called X-rays**
38.	prostatomegaly	**prostate gland enlargement**
39.	dx	**diagnosis**
40.	prostatitis	**inflammation of the prostate gland**
41.	neutered	**sexually altered**
42.	another term for neutering in male dogs	**castrated**
43.	cow	**intact female bovine that has given birth**
44.	off feed	**lack of appetite**
45.	medical term for off feed	**anorexia**
46.	teat	**nipple**
47.	udder	**milk-producing organ of ruminants and equine**
48.	quarter	**one-fourth of an udder**
49.	CMT	**California mastitis test**
50.	diagnosis	**determination of the cause of disease**
51.	mastitis	**inflammation of the mammary gland**
52.	culture	**test in which sample is collected and streaked on agar to grow any bacteria present**
53.	mare	**intact female horse 4 years or older**
54.	foaled	**gave birth to a horse**
55.	vaginal discharge	**fluid drainage from the vagina**
56.	placenta	**female organ of mammals that develops during pregnancy and joins mother and offspring for exchange of nutrients, oxygen, and waste products**
57.	retained placenta	**placenta that has not passed after parturition**
58.	postpartum	**after birth**
59.	IV	**intravenous**
60.	CBC	**complete blood count**
61.	leukocyte	**white blood cell**

CHAPTER 13

Multiple Choice

1. **a**	11. **c**
2. **c**	12. **a**
3. **b**	13. **b**
4. **d**	14. **a**
5. **d**	15. **d**
6. **c**	16. **c**
7. **d**	17. **a**
8. **b**	18. **c**
9. **c**	19. **c**
10. **a**	20. **c**

Matching

1. **e**	5. **a**
2. **c**	6. **f**
3. **d**	7. **b**
4. **g**	

Matching

8. **j**	13. **i**
9. **d**	14. **c**
10. **f**	15. **a**
11. **g**	16. **b**
12. **h**	17. **e**

Fill in the Blanks

1. **nerve or nerve tissue**
2. **layers of connective tissue enclosing the CNS**
3. **thick**
4. **knotlike mass of nerve cell bodies located outside the CNS**
5. **glue**

Spelling

1. sincope syncopy **syncope**
2. anestetic **anesthetic** anesthetick
3. **paralysis** paralisis parlysis
4. seezure siezure **seizure**
5. tosis **ptosis** ptoesis

Word Scramble

1. **neurotomy**
2. **aura**
3. **myelopathy**
4. **foramen**
5. **paraplegia**
6. **contra**
7. **epilepsy**

Crossword Puzzle

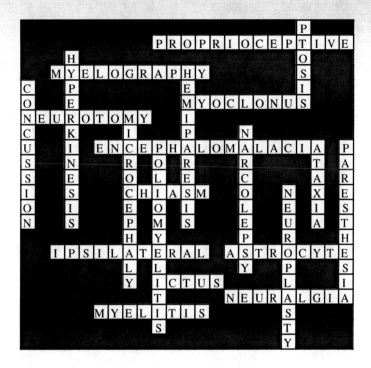

Case Studies

1.	convulsions	**sudden, violent, involuntary contractions of muscles caused by brain disturbances; also called seizures**
2.	obtunded	**depressed**
3.	neurologic	**pertaining to the nervous system**
4.	renal	**kidney**
5.	hepatic	**liver**
6.	hypoglycemia	**low blood sugar (glucose)**
7.	UA	**urinalysis**
8.	cystocentesis	**surgical puncture of the urinary bladder (to remove fluid or to inject air or contrast material)**
9.	signalment	**description of the animal [information about the animal including species, breed, age, and sexual status (intact or neutered)]**
10.	clinical	**visible, readily observed, pertaining to treatment**
11.	diagnose	**to determine the cause of disease**
12.	idiopathic	**unknown cause; disease peculiar to an individual; not likely to be seen in others**
13.	epilepsy	**recurrent seizures of nonsystemic origin**
14.	CSF tap	**removal of cerebrospinal fluid**
15.	EEG	**electroencephalogram**
16.	spayed	**female animal that is surgically altered**
17.	seizure	**sudden, violent, involuntary contraction of muscles caused by a brain disturbance**
18.	anticonvulsant	**substance that controls seizure activity**
19.	M/N	**male/neutered**
20.	lethargic	**condition of drowsiness or indifference**
21.	obese	**extremely overweight**
22.	vital signs	**parameters taken from the animal to assess its health; for example, temperature, pulse, and respiration rate**
23.	cranial nerves	**12 pairs of peripheral nerves that originate from the undersurface of the brain**
24.	CP deficit	**neurologic defect in which the animal appears not to know where its limbs are "knuckling"**

25. patellar reflexes	**automatic, involuntary response of the hindlimb to a stimulus applied to the patellar ligament ("knee jerk")**
26. hyporeflexive	**less-than-normal reflex or involuntary response to a stimulus**
27. anal	**pertaining to the anus**
28. radiographs	**records of ionizing radiation used to visualize internal body structures; also called X-rays**
29. intervertebral discs	**layers of fibrocartilage that form pads separating and cushioning the vertebrae**
30. lumbar	**loin**
31. myelography	**diagnostic study of the spinal cord after injection of contrast material**
32. myelogram	**record of the spinal cord after injection of contrast material**
33. herniated	**describes the protrusion of a body part through tissues that normally contain it**
34. disc fenestration	**removal of intervertebral disc material by perforating and scraping out its contents**

CHAPTER 14

Multiple Choice

1. **d**	11. **c**
2. **c**	12. **a**
3. **c**	13. **b**
4. **d**	14. **a**
5. **a**	15. **d**
6. **d**	16. **c**
7. **b**	17. **d**
8. **b**	18. **a**
9. **c**	19. **c**
10. **b**	20. **d**

Matching

1. **c**	5. **g**
2. **e**	6. **b**
3. **d**	7. **a**
4. **f**	

Matching

8. **f**	13. **c**
9. **e**	14. **d**
10. **i**	15. **b**
11. **j**	16. **a**
12. **g**	17. **h**

Fill in the Blanks

1. **teardrop, tear duct, or lacrimal duct**
2. **eardrum**
3. **(external) ear**
4. **eye or sight**
5. **sound or hearing**

Spelling

1. dystichiasys distechiasis **distichiasis**
2. glaukoma glawcoma **glaucoma**
3. **uveitis** uveititis uveytis
4. opague **opaque** opaiue
5. eustayshian tube eustaichian tube **eustachian tube**

Crossword Puzzles

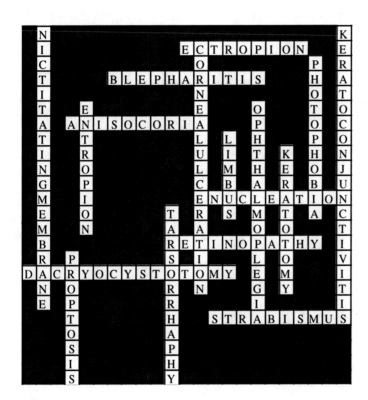

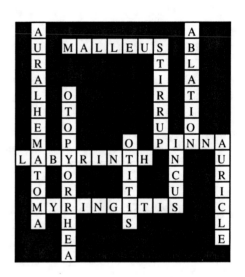

Case Studies

1.	blepharospasm	**rapid involuntary contractions of the eyelid**
2.	conjunctiva	**mucous membrane that lines the underside of each eyelid**
3.	sclera	**fibrous outer layer of the eye that maintains the shape of the eye; also called white of the eye**
4.	ocular	**pertaining to the eye**
5.	anterior chamber	**front one-third of the eyeball**
6.	iris	**pigmented muscular layer of the choroid that surrounds the pupil**
7.	tonometer	**instrument that indirectly measures intraocular pressure**
8.	OS	**left eye**
9.	mm Hg	**millimeters of mercury**
10.	OD	**right eye**
11.	uveitis	**inflammation of the uvea (iris, ciliary body, and cornea)**
12.	ocular	**pertaining to the eye**
13.	bilateral mucopurulent ocular discharge	**discharge from both eyes that contains mucus and pus**
14.	ophthalmic	**pertaining to the eye**
15.	Schirmer tear test	**diagnostic test using a graded paper strip to measure tear production**
16.	retina	**nervous tissue layer of the eye that receives images**
17.	fluorescence staining	**diagnostic test to detect corneal injury by placing dye onto the surface of the cornea**

18. blepharospasm	**rapid involuntary contraction of the eyelid**
19. entropion	**inversion or turning inward of the eyelid**
20. cornea	**transparent anterior portion of the sclera**
21. blepharoplasty	**surgical repair of the eyelid**
22. topical	**on the surface**
23. recurrent	**occurring again**
24. bilateral	**on both sides**
25. otitis externa	**inflammation of the outer or external ear**
26. cytology	**study of cells**
27. mucopurulent	**pus and mucus**
28. AU	**both ears**
29. otoscopic	**instrument to examine the ear**
30. AD	**right ear**
31. hyperemic	**excessive engorgement with blood (excessive redness)**
32. hyperkeratotic	**hypertrophy of the horny layer of skin**
33. tympanic membrane	**eardrum**
34. AS	**left ear**
35. ear ablation	**removal of the ear (or part of the ear)**

CHAPTER 15

Multiple Choice

1. **a**		11. **a**	
2. **b**		12. **b**	
3. **b**		13. **b**	
4. **c**		14. **c**	
5. **b**		15. **a**	
6. **c**		16. **c**	
7. **c**		17. **b**	
8. **c**		18. **d**	
9. **b**		19. **a**	
10. **d**		20. **b**	

Matching

1. **e**		6. **d**	
2. **f**		7. **g**	
3. **c**		8. **b**	
4. **c**		9. **a**	
5. **h**			

Matching

10. **f**		15. **g**	
11. **b**		16. **d**	
12. **a**		17. **e**	
13. **h**		18. **i**	
14. **c**		19. **j**	

Fill in the Blanks

1. **Intact**
2. **immunity**
3. **antigen**
4. **anemia**
5. **hyperemia**
6. **Anaphylaxis**
7. **allergen**
8. **oncology**
9. **lymphoma**
10. **septicemia**
11. **formation**
12. **blood**
13. **protected**
14. **blood condition**
15. **fat**

Spelling

1. erithrocyte **erythrocyte** erythrosite
2. morfology **morphology** morphlogy
3. anistocytosis **anisocytosis** anystocytosis
4. mixoma myxtoma **myxoma**
5. ostesarcoma osteosarkoma **osteosarcoma**

Crossword Puzzle

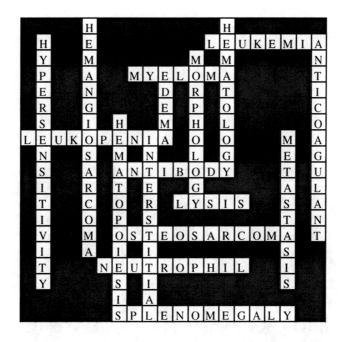

CHAPTER 16

Multiple Choice

1. **c**
2. **d**
3. **b**
4. **a**
5. **b**
6. **d**
7. **c**
8. **d**
9. **a**
10. **b**
11. **a**
12. **d**
13. **b**
14. **d**
15. **b**
16. **c**
17. **b**
18. **c**
19. **b**
20. **a**

Matching

1. **d**
2. **c or f**
3. **h**
4. **g**
5. **c or f**
6. **a**
7. **b**
8. **e**
9. **l**
10. **p**
11. **n**
12. **j**
13. **i**
14. **o**
15. **k**
16. **m**

Fill in the Blanks

1. **fire**
2. **luminous**
3. **without**
4. **heart rate**
5. **respiration rate**
6. **ventrodorsal**
7. **mediolateral oblique**
8. **dorsolateral-palmaromedial**
9. **dorsomedial-palmarolateral**
10. **dorsopalmar**

Spelling

1. virilence **virulence** virulense
2. **contagious** kontagious contagous
3. sirology sarology **serology**
4. pyrexia **pyrexa** pirexa
5. spekulum **speculum** speckulum

Crossword Puzzles

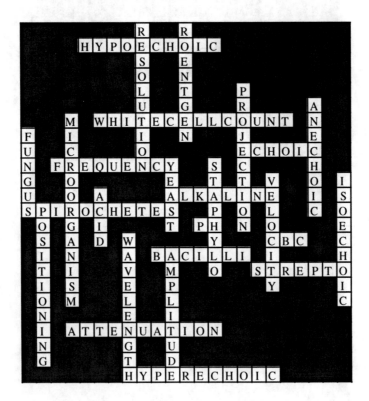

CHAPTER 17

Multiple Choice

1. **b**	11. **c**
2. **c**	12. **a**
3. **d**	13. **b**
4. **a**	14. **a**
5. **b**	15. **c**
6. **d**	16. **b**
7. **d**	17. **d**
8. **c**	18. **c**
9. **a**	19. **a**
10. **c**	20. **b**

Matching

1. **e**	6. **d**
2. **a**	7. **b**
3. **j**	8. **c**
4. **g**	9. **h**
5. **i**	10. **f**

Fill in the Blanks

1. **resect**
2. **seroma**
3. **eviscerate**
4. **fenestration**
5. **turgor**

Spelling

1. mililiter **milliliter** mililitir
2. hypercalemia hyperkallemia **hyperkalemia**
3. parental parentral **parenteral**
4. doseage doesage **dosage**
5. hydrofillic hydrophillic **hydrophilic**

Word Scramble

1. **ligation**
2. **taper**
3. **incise**
4. **cast**
5. **sling**
6. **ratchet**
7. **boxlock**
8. **rupture**
9. **enucleation**
10. **coaptation**
11. **eviscerate**
12. **transfix**

Crossword Puzzle

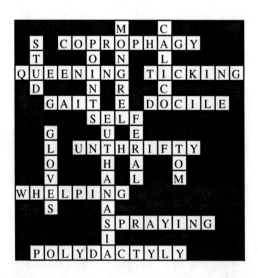

CHAPTER 18

Multiple Choice

1. **c**	11. **b**
2. **c**	12. **c**
3. **d**	13. **d**
4. **b**	14. **c**
5. **c**	15. **a**
6. **d**	16. **d**
7. **c**	17. **c**
8. **d**	18. **b**
9. **b**	19. **c**
10. **b**	20. **a**

Crossword Puzzle

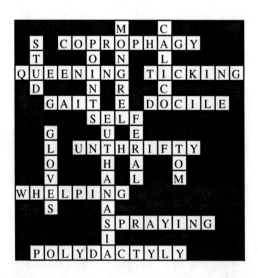

Case Studies

1.	yr	**year**
2.	F/S	**female/spayed**
3.	mandible	**lower jaw bone, the only movable bone of the skull**
4.	Hx	**history**
5.	PE	**physical examination**
6.	tachycardic	**abnormally rapid heart rate**
7.	tachypnic	**abnormally rapid breathing**
8.	rostral	**toward the nose**
9.	IV	**intravenous**
10.	caudal	**toward the tail**
11.	canine teeth	**long, pointed teeth located between the incisors and premolars; also called cuspids**
12.	antibiotics	**substances that inhibit the growth of or kill bacteria**
13.	T	**tablespoon**
14.	bid	**twice daily**
15.	PO	**orally**
16.	d	**days**
17.	wk	**week**
18.	♀	**female**
19.	DSH	**domestic shorthair (cat)**
20.	inappetence	**lacking the desire to eat**
21.	PE	**physical examination**
22.	bilateral	**on both sides**
23.	mucopurulent	**containing mucus and pus**
24.	ocular	**pertaining to the eye**
25.	nasal	**nose**
26.	T	**temperature**
27.	°F	**degrees Fahrenheit**
28.	HR	**heart rate**
29.	BPM	**beats per minute**
30.	RR	**respiration rate**
31.	min	**minute**
32.	MMs	**mucous membranes**
33.	CRT	**capillary refill time**
34.	sec	**seconds**
35.	wheeze	**abnormal, continuous, musical, whistling sound heard during inspiration or expiration; also called rhonchus**
36.	thoracic	**pertaining to the chest**
37.	auscultation	**act of listening**
38.	bronchial	**pertaining to the bronchi**
39.	URT	**upper respiratory tract**
40.	conjunctiva	**mucous membrane that covers the underside of each eyelid**
41.	edematous	**pertaining to accumulation of fluid in the intercellular space**
42.	abdomen	**area between the chest and pelvic cavities**
43.	palpated	**examined by feeling**
44.	Dx	**diagnosis**
45.	URI	**upper respiratory infection**
46.	DDx	**differential diagnosis**
47.	rhinotracheitis	**inflammation of the nose and windpipe**
48.	yr	**year**
49.	F/S	**female/spayed**
50.	DSH	**domestic shorthair (cat)**

51. stranguria	**slow or painful urination**
52. hematuria	**blood in the urine**
53. auscultated	**listened**
54. oral	**pertaining to the mouth**
55. tartar	**abnormal mineralized deposit (along with bacteria and food particles) that forms on the teeth; also called calculus**
56. gingivitis	**inflammation of the gums**
57. abdominal	**pertaining to the area between the chest and pelvic cavities**
58. palpation	**act of examining by feeling**
59. caudal	**toward the tail**
60. turgid	**swollen or congested**
61. Dx	**diagnosis**
62. cystitis	**inflammation of the urinary bladder**
63. DDx	**differential diagnosis**
64. FUS	**feline urologic syndrome (now called FLUTD)**
65. crystalluria	**crystals in the urine**
66. intact	**not sexually altered**
67. 4″	**4 inch**
68. laceration	**accidental cut into skin**
69. hemorrhage	**loss of blood (usually in a short period of time)**
70. carpus	**joint of the distal forelimb located between the radius/ulna and the metacarpals**
71. hemostasis	**to stop or control bleeding**
72. anesthetized	**provided lack of sensation**
73. ligated	**tied or strangulated**
74. sutured	**stitched**
75. OHE	**ovariohysterectomy**
76. preanesthetic	**before loss of sensation**
77. blood screen	**series of tests run on serum to assess state of an organ; also called chem panel or chem screen**
78. PCV	**packed cell volume**
79. ALT	**alanine aminotransferase (formerly SGPT)**
80. BUN	**blood urea nitrogen**
81. GLU	**glucose**
82. IV	**intravenous**
83. anesthetized	**provided lack of sensation**
84. ventral midline incision	**surgical cut along the midsagittal plane of the abdomen along the linear alba**
85. ligation	**act of tying**
86. CRT	**capillary refill time**
87. MMs	**mucous membranes**
88. tachycardic	**pertaining to an abnormally rapid heart rate**
89. hypothermic	**below normal temperature**
90. heparin	**substance that prevents clotting**
91. perianal	**surrounding the anus**
92. dermatitis	**inflammation of the skin**
93. TPR	**temperature, pulse, and respiration**
94. hx	**history**
95. tenesmus	**painful, ineffective defecation**
96. rectal palpation	**process via insertion of a gloved arm into the rectum of an animal and feeling for a specific structure**
97. anal sacs	**pair of pouches that store an oily, foul-smelling fluid secreted by the anal glands; located in the skin between the internal and external anal sphincters**
98. inspissated	**rendered dry or thick by evaporation**
99. antiseptic	**substance that kills or inhibits the growth of microorganisms on living tissue**

CHAPTER 19

Multiple Choice

1. **b**		11. **a**
2. **b**		12. **b**
3. **a**		13. **c**
4. **b**		14. **d**
5. **d**		15. **a**
6. **d**		16. **b**
7. **a**		17. **a**
8. **c**		18. **d**
9. **b**		19. **c**
10. **c**		20. **b**

Crossword Puzzle

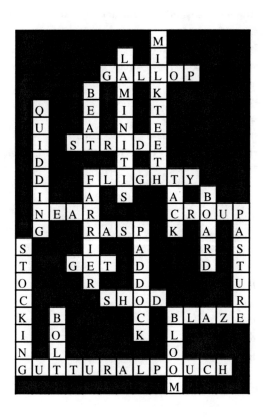

Case Studies

1. mare	**intact female horse 4 years old or older**
2. flank	**side of the body between the ribs and ilium**
3. anorexia	**lack of appetite**
4. stool	**feces; bowel movement**
5. tachycardic	**abnormally rapid heart rate**
6. hyperpnic	**abnormal increase in the rate and depth of respirations**
7. MMs	**mucous membranes**
8. CRT	**capillary refill time**
9. auscultated	**listened**
10. borborygmus	**gastrointestinal gas movement that causes a rumbling noise**
11. rectal palpation	**process via insertion of a gloved arm into the rectum of an animal and feeling for a specific structure**

12.	proximal (oral)	nearest the midline or nearest the beginning of a body structure/toward the mouth
13.	impaction	obstruction of an area usually with feed that is too dry
14.	ventral midline abdominocentsis	puncture of the abdomen along the midsagittal plane of the abdomen along the linear alba to collect fluid
15.	CBC	complete blood count
16.	peritoneal	hollow space in the abdominal cavity between the parietal and visceral peritoneums
17.	nasogastric tube	tube through the nose into the stomach
18.	NG tube	nasogastric tube
19.	analgesic	substance that relieves pain without affecting consciousness
20.	IV	intravenous
21.	colt	intact male horse (or donkey) usually under 4 years of age
22.	febrile	feverish
23.	tachycardic	abnormally rapid heart rate
24.	palpation	act of examining by feeling
25.	coronary band	junction that produces the hoof wall located between the skin and the horn of the hoof; also called the coronet
26.	pulse	rhythmic expansion and contraction of an artery produced by the pressure of blood flowing through it
27.	laminitis	inflammation of the sensitive laminae under the horny wall of the hoof
28.	radiographs	records of ionizing radiation used to visualize internal body structures; also called X-rays
29.	coffin bone	common name for the third phalanx of livestock
30.	Dx	diagnosis
31.	founder	a sequela of laminitis
32.	NSAIDs	nonsteroidal anti-inflammatory drugs
33.	farrier	person who cares for equine feet including trimming and shoeing

CHAPTER 20

Multiple Choice

1.	c	8.	b	15.	a
2.	d	9.	b	16.	b
3.	d	10.	a	17.	b
4.	b	11.	c	18.	d
5.	c	12.	d	19.	a
6.	d	13.	b	20.	b
7.	c	14.	c		

Crossword Puzzle

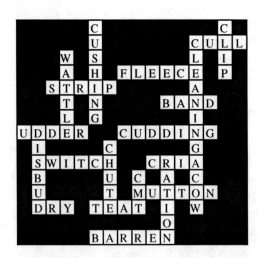

Case Studies

1.	doe	**intact female goat**
2.	dyspnea	**difficulty breathing**
3.	MMs	**mucous membranes**
4.	CRT	**capillary refill time**
5.	TPR	**temperature, pulse, and respiration**
6.	auscultated	**listened**
7.	pH	**hydrogen ion concentration, which indicates acidity or alkalinity**
8.	protozoal	**pertaining to the group of unicellular organisms that include *Giardia* and *Eimeria***
9.	rumenostomy	**creation of an artificial opening between the rumen and the body surface**
10.	L	**liter**
11.	ram	**intact male sheep**
12.	lethargy	**condition of drowsiness or indifference**
13.	anorexia	**lack of appetite**
14.	PE	**physical examination**
15.	WNL	**within normal limits**
16.	mucous membranes	**specialized form of epithelial tissue that secretes mucus**
17.	hematocrit	**percentage of erythrocytes in blood**
18.	anemic	**blood condition of less-than-normal levels of RBCs, or hemoglobin**
19.	anthelmintic	**substance that works against intestinal worms**
20.	herd	**group of cattle (and some other animals)**
21.	alopecia	**hair loss resulting in hairless patches or complete lack of hair**
22.	lesions	**pathologic change of tissue**
23.	PE	**physical examination**
24.	skin scrapings	**microscopic examinations of the skin for the presence of mites; skin is sampled by taking a scalpel blade across an area of skin that is squeezed or raised so that the sample contains a deep skin sample**
25.	microscopic examination	**viewing a sample under a microscope**
26.	mites	**arthropod that has a transparent or semitransparent body; examples include mange mites and ear mites**
27.	scabies	**contagious form of mange caused by various types of *Sarcoptes* mites**
28.	bull	**intact male bovine**
29.	paralysis	**loss of voluntary movement or immobility**
30.	anorexic	**lack or loss of appetite**
31.	ataxia	**without coordination**
32.	CBC	**complete blood count**
33.	chem panel	**series of tests run on serum to assess state of an organ; also called chemistry profile or chem screen**
34.	fecal examination	**procedure used to detect parasitic diseases of animals**
35.	eosinophilia	**elevated number of eosinophils**
36.	meningeal	**pertaining to the connective tissue surrounding the CNS**
37.	antiparasitic	**substance that works against parasites**
38.	prognosis	**prediction of the outcome of disease**

CHAPTER 21

Multiple Choice

1. **b**	8. **c**	15. **a**
2. **a**	9. **b**	16. **d**
3. **c**	10. **a**	17. **b**
4. **c**	11. **c**	18. **c**
5. **d**	12. **b**	19. **b**
6. **c**	13. **d**	20. **b**
7. **c**	14. **b**	

Crossword Puzzle

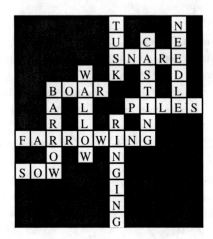

Case Studies

1.	mo	**months**
2.	barrows	**male pigs castrated when young**
3.	clinical	**pertaining to treatment**
4.	signs	**characteristic of disease that can be observed by others**
5.	purulent	**containing pus**
6.	nasal	**nose**
7.	deviation	**turning away; not straight**
8.	snout	**upper lip and apex of the nose of swine**
9.	necropsy	**examination of an animal body after death**
10.	turbinates	**scroll-like cartilages of the nasal cavity**
11.	atrophied	**wasting of tissue/decrease in cell size**
12.	asymmetrical	**dissimilarity on opposite sides**
13.	Dx	**diagnosis**
14.	rhinitis	**inflammation of the nose**
15.	yr	**year**
16.	sow	**intact female pig**
17.	dystocia	**difficulty giving birth**
18.	farrowed	**gave birth to pigs**
19.	mastitis	**inflammation of the mammary glands**
20.	agalactia	**not producing milk**
21.	uterine inertia	**condition in which uterine contractions are weak or incomplete**
22.	C-section	**cesarean section**

23. vomiting	**emesis**
24. abnormal frequency and liquidity of fecal material	**diarrhea**
25. incoordination	**ataxia**
26. elevated body temperature	**febrile or pyrexic**
27. termination of pregnancy	**abortion**
28. wild	**feral**

CHAPTER 22

Multiple Choice

1. **b**	11. **c**
2. **a**	12. **b**
3. **d**	13. **d**
4. **c**	14. **a**
5. **b**	15. **d**
6. **d**	16. **c**
7. **b**	17. **b**
8. **a**	18. **a**
9. **d**	19. **d**
10. **b**	20. **b**

Crossword Puzzle

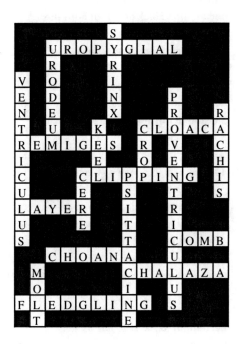

Case Studies

1.	neonatal	newborn animal
2.	radiograph	record of ionizing radiation used to visualize internal body structures; also called X-ray
3.	crop	esophageal enlargement that stores, moistens, and softens food in some birds
4.	proventriculus	elongated, spindle-shaped glandular stomach of birds
5.	ingluviotomy	incision into the crop (also known as cropotomy)
6.	endoscope	tubelike instrument with lights and refracting mirrors that is used to examine the body or organs internally
7.	anesthesia	lack of sensation
8.	thorax	chest area
9.	thoracic inlet	entrance route into the thorax (located cranially)
10.	cm	centimeter
11.	subcutaneously	under the skin
12.	rostral	toward the nose
13.	diagnoses	determinations of the cause of disease
14.	neoplasia	process of any abnormal new growth of tissue in which the multiplication of cells is uncontrolled, more rapid than normal, and progressive
15.	lipoma	benign growth of fat cells
16.	xanthoma	nodule in skin due to lipid deposits
17.	fine needle aspirate (FNA)	insertion of a needle to obtain a tissue sample by the suction applied from a syringe
18.	hypothyroidism	less-than-normal amounts of thyroid hormone or thyroid gland activity
19.	flock	group of birds
20.	cockerels	immature male chickens
21.	pullets	immature female chickens
22.	anorexic	pertaining to lack or loss of appetite
23.	emaciated	marked wasting or excessive leanness
24.	droppings	composite of feces and urine in birds
25.	asymptomatic	without clinical signs of disease
26.	layers	chickens raised for egg production
27.	brooder	housing unit for rearing birds after hatching
28.	cage operation	method of raising chickens in which the hens are kept in confinement as they produce eggs
29.	ostrich	large, flightless bird native to Africa that is the largest ratite (can weigh over 400 pounds) and may be black, blue, or red
30.	flock	group of birds
31.	chicks	young ratite (usually less than 6 months of age)
32.	paralysis	loss of voluntary movement or immobility
33.	torticollis	contracted state of the cervical muscles producing torsion of the neck
34.	ataxia	without coordination
35.	opisthotonus	tetanic spasm in which the head and tail are bent dorsally and the back is arched
36.	mortality	ratio of disease animals that die to diseased animals
37.	histological	pertaining to the study of tissue
38.	serology	laboratory study of serum and the reactions of antigens and antibodies

CHAPTER 23

Multiple Choice

1. **a**	8. **c**	15. **a**
2. **c**	9. **c**	16. **d**
3. **b**	10. **d**	17. **d**
4. **b**	11. **a**	18. **b**
5. **b**	12. **c**	19. **c**
6. **b**	13. **b**	20. **c**
7. **c**	14. **b**	

Crossword Puzzle

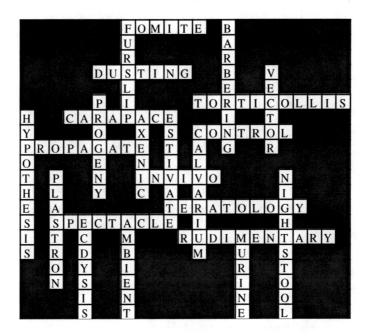

Case Studies

1.	lethargy	**condition of drowsiness or indifference**
2.	ataxia	**incoordination**
3.	PE	**physical examination**
4.	hyperparathyroidism	**more than normal levels of parathormone or parathyroid gland activity**
5.	metabolic	**processes involved in the body's use of nutrients**
6.	radiographs	**records of ionizing radiation used to visualize internal body structures; also called X-rays**
7.	serum	**liquefied portion of blood with clotting proteins removed**
8.	chemistry profile	**series of tests run on serum to assess state of an organ; also called chem panel or chem screen**
9.	hypocalcemia	**less-than-normal levels of blood calcium**
10.	hypoproteinemia	**less-than-normal levels of blood protein**
11.	tympanic membrane	**eardrum**
12.	laterally	**toward the side**
13.	oral	**pertaining to the mouth**
14.	stomatitis	**inflammation of the mouth**
15.	plaques	**small, differentiated, raised area on a body surface**

16. mucosa   **another term for mucous membrane**

17. diagnosis   **determination of the cause of disease**

18. otitis media   **inflammation of the middle ear**

19. hypovitaminosis   **abnormal condition of less-than-normal amounts of vitamins**

20. abscess   **localized collection of pus**

21. lanced   **incised with a scalpel or pointed blade**

22. debrided   **removed foreign material and devitalized or contaminated tissue**

23. cytology   **study of cells**

24. squamous   **flat, platelike**

25. metaplasia   **change in mature cells to an abnormal form**

26. alopecia   **hair loss resulting in hairless patches or complete lack of hair**

27. dorsal lumbar   **area of the back located between the loin and tail**

28. dysuria   **difficulty urinating**

29. ectoparasites   **parasites that live on the surface of the body**

30. dermatophytosis   **abnormal skin condition with superficial fungus**

31. atopy   **hypersensitivity reaction in animals involving pruritus with secondary dermatitis; commonly called allergies**

32. cystitis   **inflammation of the urinary bladder**

33. urolithiasis   **condition of urinary bladder stones**

34. dx   **diagnosis**

35. hyperadrenocorticism   **condition of excessive adrenal cortex production of glucocorticoid; also called Cushing's disease**

36. hyperplasia   **abnormal increase in the number of normal cells that are in normal arrangement in a tissue**

37. neoplasia   **process of any abnormal new growth of tissue in which the multiplication of cells is uncontrolled, more rapid than normal, and progressive**

38. cessation   **act of stopping**

39. prostatic hyperplasia   **abnormal increase in the number of normal prostatic cells that are in normal arrangement in a tissue**

40. excision   **process of cutting out**

41. midshaft   **midway between the epiphyses of a long bone**

42. spiral   **winding**

43. femoral fx   **break (fracture) of the thigh bone**

44. diagnosed   **determined the cause of disease**

45. radiographs   **records of ionizing radiation used to visualize internal body structures; also called X-rays**

46. coaptation   **act of approximating**

47. splinting   **putting on a rigid or flexible appliance for fixation of movable or displaced parts**

48. fx   **fracture**

49. inhalant anesthetic   **gas form of a substance that produces lack of sensation**

50. viable   **livable**

51. vascular   **pertaining to vessels (blood)**

52. amputation   **removal of all or part of a body part**

53. ambulated   **moved (walked)**

54. hematuria   **blood in the urine**

55. pollakiuria   **frequent urination**

56. hx   **history**

57. BAR   **bright, alert, responsive**

58. WNL   **within normal limits**

59. palpation   **act of examining by feeling**

60. vocalization   **act of making sound**

61. cystocentesis   **surgical puncture of the urinary bladder (to remove fluid)**

62. UA   **urinalysis**

63. erythrocytes   **red blood cells**

64.	leukocytes	**white blood cells**
65.	crystals	**angular solid of definitive form**
66.	urolith	**urinary bladder stone**
67.	radiographs	**records of ionizing radiation used to visualize internal body structures; also called X-rays**
68.	radiopaque	**quality of appearing white or light gray on an X-ray**
69.	cystotomy	**incision into the urinary bladder**
70.	pruritus	**itchiness**
71.	dorsal	**toward the back**
72.	dorsal cervical region	**back area located in the neck region**
73.	debris	**dead or foreign material**
74.	ectoparasitic	**parasite that lives on body surfaces**
75.	topically	**on a surface**
76.	parasiticide	**substance that kills parasites**
77.	interscapular	**between the shoulder blades (scapula)**
78.	conjunctivitis	**inflammation of the mucous membrane that lines the underside of each eyelid**
79.	sinusitis	**inflammation of a sinus**
80.	nares	**nostrils**
81.	nasal	**nose**
82.	etiologic	**disease-causing**
83.	antibiotic	**substance that inhibits the growth of or kills bacteria**
84.	PO	**orally (per os)**
85.	chronic	**long course, progressive onset, persistent for a long time**

PART IV

CROSSWORD
PUZZLES

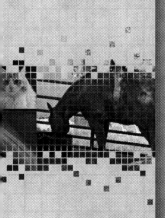

CHAPTER 1 PREFIXES AND SUFFIXES

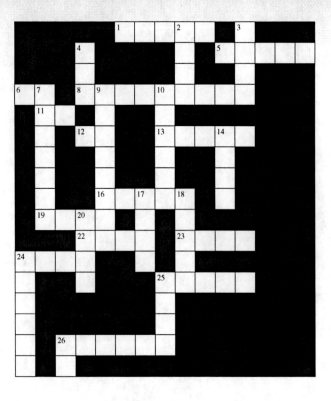

Across

1. prefix meaning between
5. suffix for to surgically create a new opening
6. suffix for structure
8. suffix for abnormal hardening
11. prefix meaning opposite of towards
12. prefix meaning without
13. prefix meaning excessive
16. prefix for excessive
19. prefix meaning against
22. suffix for an abnormal condition
23. prefix for less than normal
24. suffix meaning a record of
25. suffix for disease
26. suffix for surgical removal

Down

2. prefix meaning outside
3. suffix for inflammation
4. prefix meaning opposite of good
7. suffix for abnormal softening
9. suffix meaning surgical puncture to remove fluid
10. suffix for bursting forth
14. prefix meaning inside
17. prefix meaning after
18. suffix for discharge
20. suffix for cutting into
24. suffix meaning a procedure that records
25. suffix meaning to suture to stabilize
26. prefix meaning outside

CHAPTER 1 PREFIXES AND SUFFIXES ANSWERS

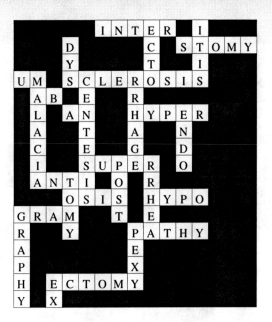

CHAPTER 2 ORGAN COMBINING FORMS

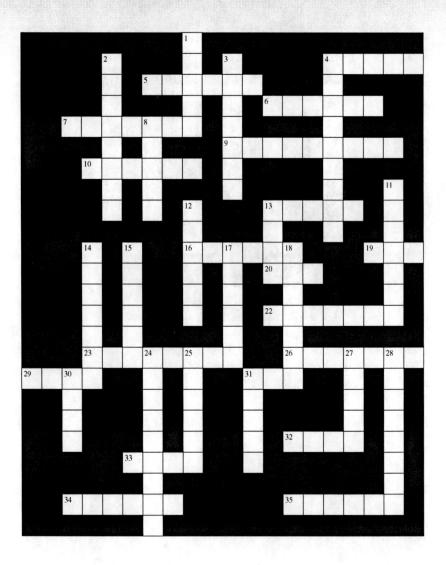

Across

4. bone
5. stomach
6. kidney
7. larynx
9. brain
10. lungs
13. thymus
16. spleen
19. ear
20. mouth
22. cartilage
23. esophagus
26. skin

29. vein
31. muscle
32. large intestine
33. blood
34. liver
35. heart

Down

1. urinary bladder
2. pharynx
3. ureters
4. eye
8. nerves
11. urethra

12. fascia
13. tendon
14. trachea
15. small intestine
17. lymph vessel, fluid, or node
18. testes
24. pancreas
25. joint
27. uterus
28. tonsil
30. nose or nares
31. spinal cord

CHAPTER 2 ORGAN COMBINING FORMS ANSWERS

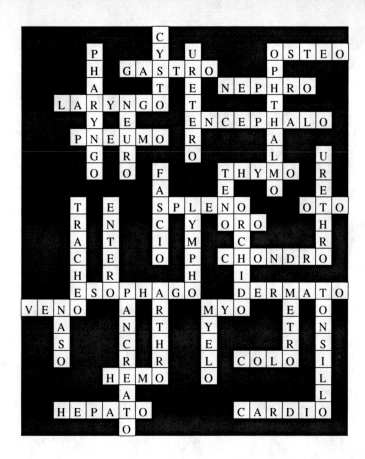

CHAPTER 3 STRUCTURAL SUPPORT TERMS

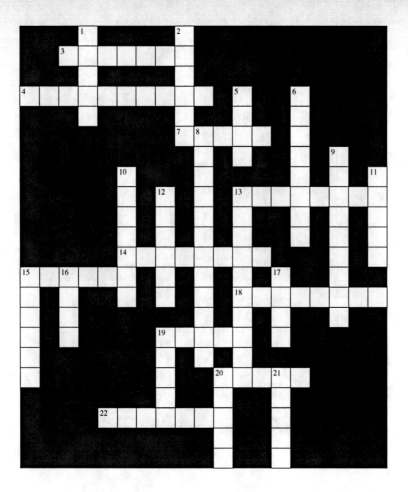

Across

3. rounded projection (that articulates with another bone)
4. projecting part
7. sharp projection
13. pulley shaped structure in which other structures pass or articulate
14. surface projection
15. groove
18. opening
19. smooth area
20. high projection or border projection
22. hole

Down

1. small pit
2. passage or opening
5. toothlike structure
6. small, rounded surface projection
8. projecting part
9. rounded projection (distal end of tibia and fibula)
10. projection
11. branch or smaller structure given off by a larger structure
12. thin flat plate
13. broad, flat projection (on femur)
15. seam
16. low projection or ridge
17. major protrusion
19. trench or hollow depressed area
20. tunnel
21. space or cavity

CHAPTER 3 STRUCTURAL SUPPORT TERMS ANSWERS

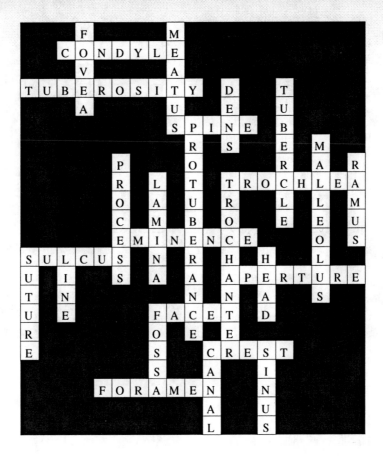

CHAPTER 4 HEAD TO TOE (ANIMAL PARTS)

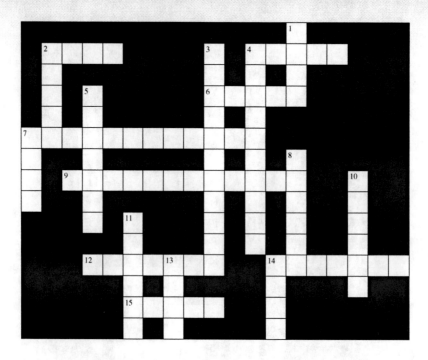

Across

2. protrusion of the ischium bones just lateral to the base of the tail in ruminants
4. protrusion of the wing of the ilium on the dorsolateral area of ruminants
6. side of the body between the ribs and ilium
7. joint between the long and short pastern bones (phalanx I and II respectively) in ungulates (an ungulate is an animal with hooves)
9. metacarpophalangeal and metatarsophalangeal joint in ungulates
12. mass of connective tissue, muscle, and fat covering the cranioventral part of the ruminant chest between the forelegs
14. accessory claw of the ruminant foot that projects caudally from fetlock
15. upper margin of the neck

Down

1. tarsal joint
2. projecting part of the ear lying outside the head; the auricle
3. joint between the short pastern and coffin bones (phalanx I and II respectively) in ungulates
4. circumference of the chest just caudal to the shoulders and cranial to the back
5. region over the dorsum where the neck joins the thorax and where the dorsal margins of the scapula lie just below the skin
7. top of the head; the occiput
8. femorotibial and femoropatellar joint in quadrupeds
10. the two nostrils (including the skin and fascia) and the muscles of the upper and lower lip
11. tuft of hair at the end of the tail
13. the carpus in ungulates
14. amputation of the tail

CHAPTER 4 HEAD TO TOE (ANIMAL PARTS) ANSWERS

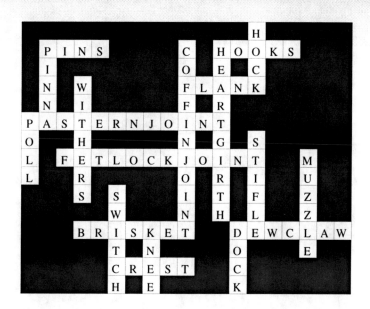

CHAPTER 5 ANIMAL NAMES

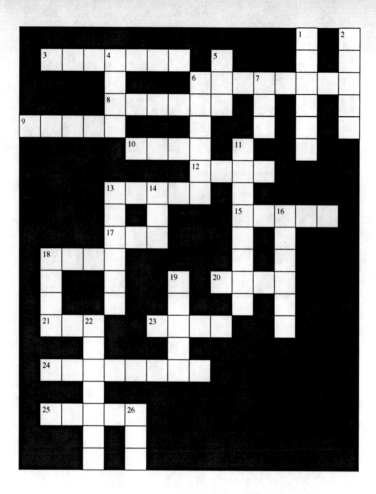

Across

3. castrated llama
6. immature male chicken
8. group of geese
9. caprines
10. male horse under 4 years
12. felines
13. female dog
15. castrated rabbit
17. male ovine
18. male swine
20. young horse
21. young goat
23. group of bovine
24. giving birth to a ferret or rabbit
25. ovine

Down

1. equines
2. female horse under 4 years
4. canines
5. female rabbit or goat
6. group of eggs
7. young ferret or rabbit
11. male horse over 4 years old
13. male swine castrated when young
14. male turkey
16. immature female chicken
18. male rabbit or goat
19. female cat
22. burros
26. young mouse or rat

CHAPTER 5 ANIMAL NAMES ANSWERS

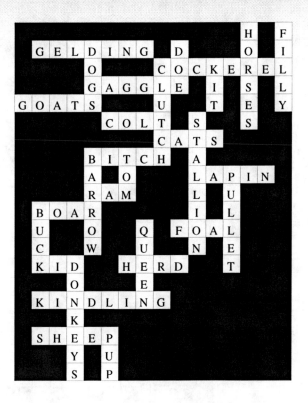

CHAPTER 6 DIGESTIVE ORGANS AND DISEASES

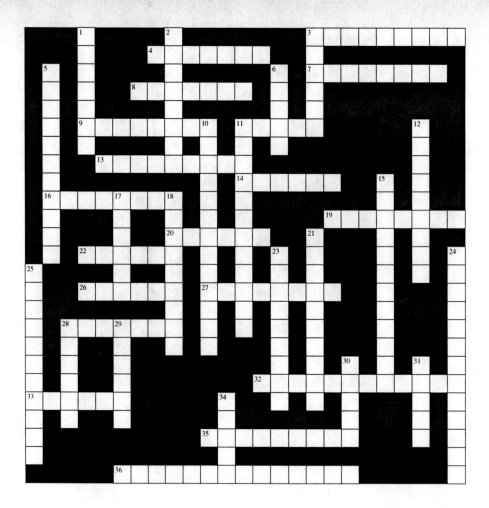

Across

3. most cranial compartment of the ruminant stomach
4. middle portion of small intestine
7. general ill health and malnutrition
8. throat
9. excessive salivation
11. distal or aboral portion of the small intestine
13. collapsible muscular tube that leads from the oral cavity to the stomach
14. roof of the mouth
16. proximal or oral portion of the small intestine
19. gland that secretes digestive juices as well as hormones
20. combining form for tongue
22. black stools containing digested blood
26. combining form for stomach
27. combining form for nourishment
28. combining form for mouth
32. hairball
33. another term for dental calculus
35. inflammation of the tongue
36. enter/o is the combining form for this GI organ

Down

1. abnormal accumulation of fluid in tissues or a body cavity
2. stonelike fecal mass
3. distal or aboral portion of the large intestine
5. organ that stores bile
6. organ that produces bile
10. abnormally large esophagus
11. process of rendering dry or thick by evaporation
12. difficulty defecating
15. inability to control
17. benign tumor arising from periodontal mucous membranes
18. abnormally large colon
21. excessive gas formation in the GI tract
23. cheek teeth found between canine teeth and molars
24. impaired uptake of nutrients from the intestine
25. excessive loss of body water or fluid
28. diarrhea in livestock
29. most caudally located cheek teeth
30. rounded mass of food, large pharmaceutical preparation, or to give something rapidly
31. severe abdominal pain
34. part of large intestine located between the cecum and rectum

CHAPTER 6 DIGESTIVE ORGANS AND DISEASES ANSWERS

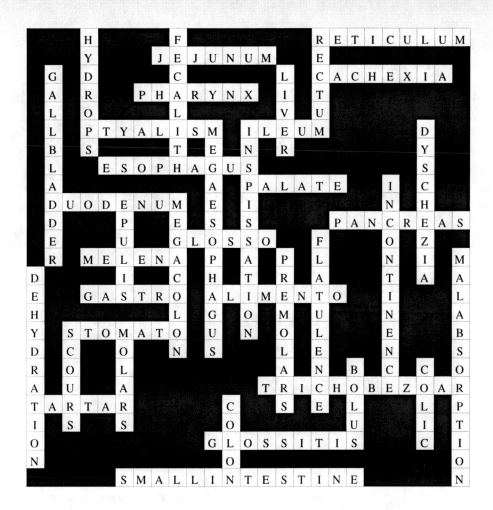

CHAPTER 14 EYES AND EARS

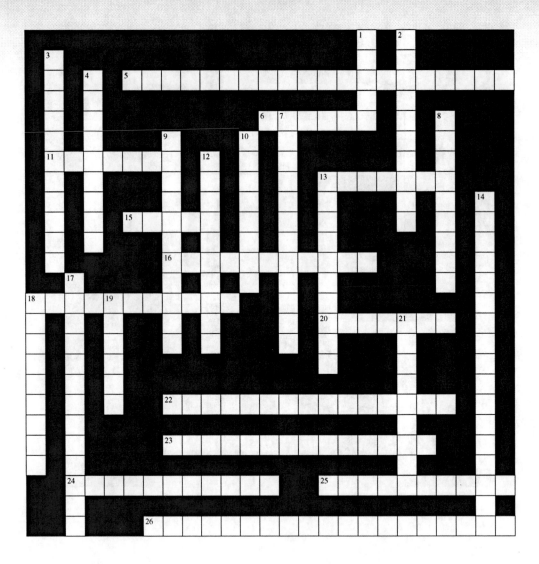

Across

5. inflammation of the cornea and mucous membranes that line the eyelid
6. inflammation of the ear
11. another term for pinna
13. another term for stapes
15. external portion of the ear
16. intolerance of light
18. removal of the eyeball
20. another term for hammer
22. incision into the lacrimal sac
23. paralysis of the eye muscles
24. pus discharge from the ear
25. inflammation of the ear drum
26. another term for third eyelid

Down

1. another term for anvil
2. condition of unequal pupil size
3. inflammation of the eyelid
4. another term for the inner ear
7. suturing together of the eyelids
8. displacement of the eye from the orbit
9. any disorder of the retina
10. removal of a part by cutting
12. incision into the cornea
13. disorder in which the eyes are not directed in a parallel manner
14. surface depression on the cornea
17. collection of blood on the outer ear
18. eversion of the eyelid
19. corneoscleral junction
21. inversion of the eyelid

CHAPTER 14 EYES AND EARS ANSWERS

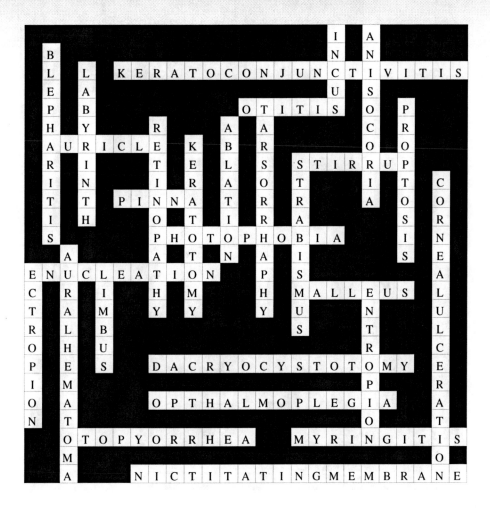

CHAPTER 15 HEMATOLOGIC, LYMPHATIC, AND IMMUNE SYSTEM TERMS

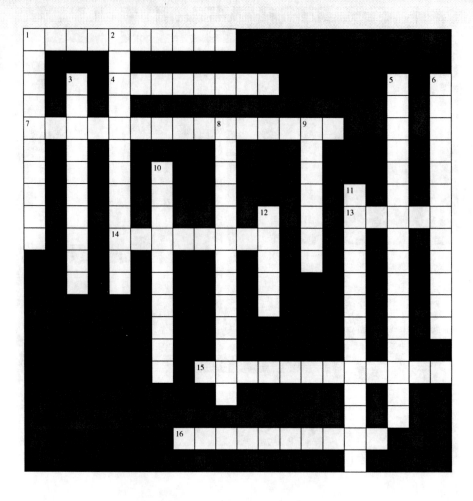

Across

1. pathogenic growth distant from the primary disease site
4. abnormal increase in the number of malignant WBCs
7. malignant neoplasm of vascular tissue
13. accumulation of fluid in the intercellular space
14. disease-fighting protein produced by the body in response to the presence of a foreign substance
15. pertaining to the spaces within a tissue or organ
16. abnormal decrease in the number of WBCs

Down

1. study of form
2. enlargement of the spleen
3. study of blood
5. another term for allergy
6. malignant neoplasm of bone
8. substance that prevents clotting
9. malignant neoplasm of bone marrow
10. another name for polymorphonuclear leukocyte
11. formation of blood
12. destruction or breakdown

CHAPTER 15 HEMATOLOGIC, LYMPHATIC, AND IMMUNE SYSTEM TERMS ANSWERS

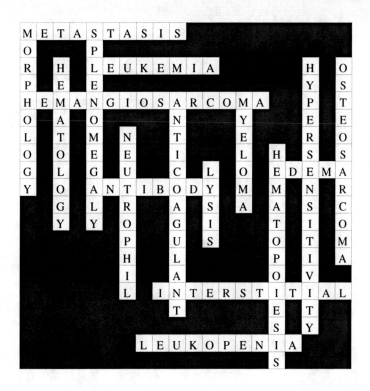

CHAPTER 16 LABORATORY AND RADIOGRAPHIC TERMS

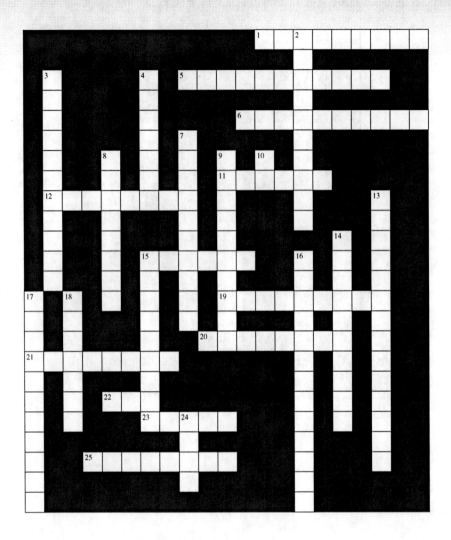

Across

1. intensity of an ultrasound wave
5. specified body position and the part of the body closest to the film
6. tissue that reflects more sound back to the transducer than the surrounding tissues; appears bright
11. ultrasound property of producing adequate levels of reflections (echoes) when sound waves are returned to the transducer and displayed
12. high pH property
15. eukaryotic organism without chlorophyll
19. tissue that has the same ultrasonic appearance as that of the surrounding tissue
20. ultrasonic term for when waves are transmitted to deeper tissue and none are reflected back
21. international unit of radiation
22. diagnostic evaluation of blood to determine the number of RBC, WBC, and thrombocytes per cubic milliliter of blood
23. budding form of fungus
25. speed at which something travels through an object

Down

2. path of the X-ray beam
3. loss of intensity of the ultrasound beam as it travels through tissue
4. rod-shaped bacteria
7. length that a wave must travel in one cycle
8. combining form for grapelike clusters
9. ability to separately identify different structures on the radiograph or ultrasound
10. concentration of hydrogen ions
13. number of leukocytes per cubic milliliter of blood
14. tissue that reflects less sound back to the transducer than the surrounding tissues; appears dark
15. number of cycles per unit of time
16. microscopic living organism
17. spiral-shaped bacteria
18. combining form for chain
24. low pH property

CHAPTER 16 LABORATORY AND RADIOGRAPHIC TERMS ANSWERS

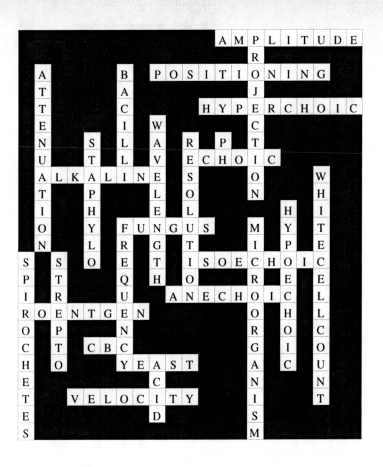

PART V

[CASE STUDIES]

TESTING MEDICAL TERM OR ABBREVIATION KNOWLEDGE

Provide the Medical Term or Abbreviation for the Boldfaced Words in Each Case Study

Case Study 1

An eight-year-old **female spayed domestic shorthair** cat was seen at the clinic for a history of **itchiness** and **hair loss resulting in bald patches**. The cat was current on vaccinations and had no other health problems. The cat shared a household with no other cat that was losing hair. **Physical examination** revealed normal vital signs, a normal **examination by feeling** of the **area between the chest cavity and pelvis**, and normal **examination by listening**. The alopecia was noted along the "**back**" midline in the **loin** area. No skin abnormalities were seen. Differential diagnoses for alopecia in cats include infection, **allergies**, **external bugs**, **hormonal diseases**, and behavioral problems. The cat was hospitalized for further testing, including skin scrapes, **within-the-skin** skin testing, and blood collection.

1. female spayed _____
2. domestic shorthair _____
3. itchiness _____
4. hair loss resulting in bald patches _____
5. physical examination _____
6. examination by feeling _____
7. area between the chest cavity and pelvis _____
8. examination by listening _____
9. "back" _____
10. loin _____
11. allergies _____
12. external bugs _____
13. hormonal diseases _____
14. within-the-skin _____

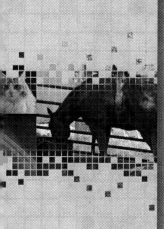

93

Case Study 2

A 5-yr-old M/N black poodle is presented to the clinic with exercise intolerance. Upon PE, it is observed that the dog is **indifferent**. Upon palpation, it is noted that there is an **abnormal accumulation of fluid in the abdomen**. The chest is **listened to**, and an **abnormal swishing sound** is heard. A cardiac workup is completed (EKG, radiographs, and echocardiogram), and the dog is dx'd with mitral valve prolapse. The mitral valve prolapse is advanced, which has caused **enlargement of the heart**.

1. indifferent _____
2. abnormal accumulation of fluid in the abdomen _____
3. listened to _____
4. abnormal swishing sound _____
5. enlargement of the heart _____

Case Study 3

A 3-yr-old F/S DSH presented to the clinic with **blood in the urine** and **difficulty urinating**. Urine was collected by **inserting a needle into the urinary bladder and withdrawing urine** and a **test on the urine involving breakdown of the urine components** was performed. The cat was dx'd with cystitis and put on antibiotics. After 2 months of treatment with various antibiotics and urinary acidifiers, radiographs, and culture and sensitivity testing of the urine, the cat still has signs of cystitis. The cat was admitted to the clinic and an ultrasound was performed to rule out **urinary bladder stones**. The ultrasound revealed that there were no stones in the urinary bladder and therapy was continued. A test on the urine was repeated 1 week after the ultrasound and the cat was responding to therapy. Within another week the cat was greatly improved and the owner was happy.

1. blood in the urine _____
2. difficulty urinating _____
3. inserting a needle into the urinary bladder and withdrawing urine _____
4. test on the urine involving breakdown of the urine components _____
5. urinary bladder stones _____

TESTING DEFINITION KNOWLEDGE

Provide Definitions, Medical Terms, or Abbreviations for the List of Terms Following Each Case Study

Case Study 4

A F/S dog was brought to the clinic with severe **dyspnea**. The veterinarian **auscultated** the **thoracic** area and determined that the dog had **tachycardia** and **tachypnea**. Upon further testing of the dog (via **radiographs**), the veterinarian determined that the dog had **pneumothorax** and recommended placement of a chest tube to relieve the dyspnea.

1. dyspnea _____
2. auscultated _____
3. thoracic _____
4. tachycardia _____
5. tachypnea _____
6. radiographs _____
7. pneumothorax _____

Case Study 5

A 5-**yr**-old Holstein is **off feed**, has pasty stool, and is **lethargic**. The veterinarian does a **PE** and determines **T** = 100°F, **HR** = 36 **bpm**, and **RR** = 24 breaths/min. The veterinarian **auscults** the **thoracic** and **abdominal** cavities. During the PE, the cow goes down and will not get up. Because the cow had just **freshened**, **milk fever** is suspected. The cow is treated with **IV** calcium and rises shortly after treatment. The veterinarian discussed nutritional management with the farmer.

1. yr _____
2. off feed _____
3. lethargic _____
4. PE _____
5. T _____
6. HR _____
7. bpm _____
8. RR _____
9. auscults _____
10. thoracic _____
11. abdominal _____
12. freshened _____
13. milk fever _____
14. IV _____

Case Study 6

An 8-**yr**-old **mare** is presented to the clinic **c̄ dyspnea**. Her **MMs** are pale, and the veterinarian suspects **hypoxia**. The veterinarian **auscults** the **thoracic** cavity, especially focusing on whether fluid is present in the chest. **Percussion** reveals a fluid line. The veterinarian also determines that the horse is **bradycardic** and has harsh lung sounds. The veterinarian suspects **pleuritis**.

1. yr _____
2. mare _____
3. c̄ _____
4. dyspnea _____
5. MMs _____
6. hypoxia _____
7. auscults _____
8. thoracic _____
9. percussion _____
10. bradycardic _____
11. pleuritis _____

Case Study 7

A 14-**yr**-old Manx cat has **alopecia**, is **anorexic**, and has been losing weight. On **PE**, the **otoscopic** exam was normal, **auscultation** with a **stethoscope** was normal, and **palpation** was normal. A **CBC** and chemistry panel (with a T_4 measurement) were run on a jugular blood sample. A **UA** was performed on a **cystocentesis** samples, and **hematuria** was observed upon gross examination of the urine. UA results confirmed **cystitis**, and urine was cultured to determine the causative agent of the cystitis. Both **V/D** and **lateral radiographs** were taken. Fungal cultures and skin scrapings were performed to assess the cause of the alopecia. **Antibiotics** were prescribed **po** pending results of the urine culture and skin tests.

1. yr _____
2. alopecia _____
3. anorexic _____
4. PE _____
5. otoscopic _____
6. auscultation _____
7. stethoscope _____
8. palpation _____
9. CBC _____
10. T_4 _____
11. UA _____
12. cystocentesis _____
13. hematuria _____
14. cystitis _____
15. V/D _____
16. lateral _____
17. radiographs _____
18. antibiotics _____
19. po _____

Answers to Case Study 1

1. female spayed	**F/S**	
2. domestic shorthair	**DSH**	
3. itchiness	**pruritus**	
4. hair loss resulting in bald patches	**alopecia**	
5. physical examination	**PE**	
6. examination by feeling	**palpation**	
7. area between the chest cavity and pelvis	**abdomen**	
8. examination by listening	**auscultation**	
9. "back"	**dorsal**	
10. loin	**lumbar**	
11. allergies	**lesions**	
12. external bugs	**ectoparasites**	
13. hormonal diseases	**endocrinopathies**	
14. within-the-skin	**intradermal**	

Answers to Case Study 2

1. indifferent	**lethargic**
2. abnormal accumulation of fluid in the abdomen	**ascites**
3. listened to	**auscultated**
4. abnormal swishing sound	**murmur**
5. enlargement of the heart	**cardiomegaly**

Answers to Case Study 3

1. blood in the urine	**hematuria**
2. difficulty urinating	**dysuria**
3. inserting a needle into the urinary bladder and withdrawing urine	**cystocentesis**
4. test on the urine involving breakdown of the urine components	**urinalysis, or UA**
5. urinary bladder stones	**urinary calculi, uroliths, or cystoliths**

Answers to Case Study 4

1. dyspnea	**difficulty breathing**
2. auscultated	**examined by listening**
3. thoracic	**pertaining to the chest**
4. tachycardia	**abnormally rapid heart rate**
5. tachypnea	**abnormally rapid breathing**
6. radiographs	**X-rays**
7. pneumothorax	**abnormal accumulation of gas or air in the chest cavity**

Answers to Case Study 5

1. yr	**year**
2. off feed	**anorexic; common term for not eating**
3. lethargic	**indifferent**
4. PE	**physical examination**
5. T	**temperature**
6. HR	**heart rate**
7. bpm	**beats per minute**
8. RR	**respiratory rate**

9. auscults	**examines by listening**
10. thoracic	**pertaining to the chest**
11. abdominal	**pertaining to the area between the chest cavity and pelvis**
12. freshened	**given birth to a dairy animal; in cattle, may be referred to as calving**
13. milk fever	**hypocalcemic metabolic disorder of ruminants seen in late pregnancy or early lactation; also called parturient paresis**
14. IV	**intravenous**

Answers for Case Study 6

1. yr	**year**
2. mare	**intact female horse over 4 years of age**
3. c̄	**with**
4. dyspnea	**difficulty breathing**
5. MMs	**mucous membranes**
6. hypoxia	**less-than-normal levels of oxygen**
7. auscults	**examines by listening**
8. thoracic	**pertaining to the chest**
9. percussion	**examination by tapping an area and listening for changes in sound**
10. bradycardic	**describes an abnormally slow heart rate**
11. pleuritis	**inflammation of the pleura (membrane lining the lungs)**

Answers to Case Study 7

1. yr	**year**
2. alopecia	**hair loss resulting in areas of baldness**
3. anorexic	**referring to not eating**
4. PE	**physical examination**
5. otoscopic	**pertaining to examination of the ear using an instrument**
6. auscultation	**act of examining by listening**
7. stethoscope	**instrument used to listen (stetho/o means chest)**
8. palpation	**act of examining by feeling**
9. CBC	**complete blood count**
10. T_4	**one of the thyroid hormones**
11. UA	**urinalysis**
12. cystocentesis	**puncture of the urinary bladder with a needle to collect urine**
13. hematuria	**blood in the urine**
14. cystitis	**inflammation of the urinary bladder**
15. V/D	**ventral/dorsal**
16. lateral	**pertaining to the side**
17. radiographs	**X-rays**
18. antibiotics	**chemicals that kill or inhibit the growth of bacteria**
19. po	**per os; orally**